T0100264

COMPUTATIONAL METABOLOMICS

METABOLIC DISEASES - LABORATORY AND CLINICAL RESEARCH

Additional books in this series can be found on Nova's website under the Series tab.

Additional E-books in this series can be found on Nova's website under the E-book tab.

MATHEMATICS RESEARCH DEVELOPMENTS

Additional books in this series can be found on Nova's website under the Series tab.

Additional E-books in this series can be found on Nova's website under the E-book tab.

METABOLIC DISEASES - LABORATORY AND CLINICAL RESEARCH

COMPUTATIONAL METABOLOMICS

NABIL SEMMAR

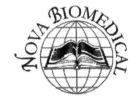

Nova Biomedical Books
New York

Copyright © 2011 by Nova Science Publishers, Inc.

All rights reserved. No part of this book may be reproduced, stored in a retrieval system or transmitted in any form or by any means: electronic, electrostatic, magnetic, tape, mechanical photocopying, recording or otherwise without the written permission of the Publisher.

For permission to use material from this book please contact us:
Telephone 631-231-7269; Fax 631-231-8175
Web Site: http://www.novapublishers.com

NOTICE TO THE READER
The Publisher has taken reasonable care in the preparation of this book, but makes no expressed or implied warranty of any kind and assumes no responsibility for any errors or omissions. No liability is assumed for incidental or consequential damages in connection with or arising out of information contained in this book. The Publisher shall not be liable for any special, consequential, or exemplary damages resulting, in whole or in part, from the readers' use of, or reliance upon, this material. Any parts of this book based on government reports are so indicated and copyright is claimed for those parts to the extent applicable to compilations of such works.

Independent verification should be sought for any data, advice or recommendations contained in this book. In addition, no responsibility is assumed by the publisher for any injury and/or damage to persons or property arising from any methods, products, instructions, ideas or otherwise contained in this publication.

This publication is designed to provide accurate and authoritative information with regard to the subject matter covered herein. It is sold with the clear understanding that the Publisher is not engaged in rendering legal or any other professional services. If legal or any other expert assistance is required, the services of a competent person should be sought. FROM A DECLARATION OF PARTICIPANTS JOINTLY ADOPTED BY A COMMITTEE OF THE AMERICAN BAR ASSOCIATION AND A COMMITTEE OF PUBLISHERS.

Additional color graphics may be available in the e-book version of this book.

Library of Congress Cataloging-in-Publication Data

Semmar, Nabil.
 Computational metabolomics / author, Nabil Semmar.
   p. ; cm.
 Includes bibliographical references and index.
  ISBN 978-1-61761-608-2 (hardcover)
 1. Metabolites. I. Title.
 [DNLM: 1. Metabolomics--methods. 2. Computational Biology--methods. QU 120]
  QP171.S46 210
  570.285--dc22
                        2010033045

Published by Nova Science Publishers, Inc. † New York

CONTENTS

PREFACE

Metabolism represents a complex system characterized by a high variability in metabolites' structures, concentrations and regulation ratios. Such variability is observed at different metabolic scales going from metabolites to metabolic profiles via chemical reactions and metabolic pathways, and under static or dynamic aspects. These components vary quantitatively and qualitatively by different processes including apparition-disappearence, increase-decrease in concentration and regulation levels, variation of local enzymatic activity or global pathway expression, etc. These different processes lead to different structural, functional and evolutive states of the metabolic system. Analysis of the different metabolic states and their control processes (generating or governing) require the use of different mathematical tools which provide appropriate solutions to different questions on the system:

Complex topologies of metabolic systems can be mathematically structured by using appropriate matrices giving separated information on the different components of system. These matrices give invariant or variant characteristics of the system: Stoichiometric matrix characterizes *a priori* the system by all its chemical reactions (invariant characteristics), and is used as a basis to predict the states of adjustable (variant) parameters (e.g. metabolic flux distributions) in the system. On the other hand, concentration matrix characterizes *a posteriori* a metabolic system by variant parameters consisting of different metabolites analysed in different individuals (subjects). From such a matrix, a correlation analysis can be applied to highlight different relationships between metabolites' levels. This helps to understand the organization and relative behaviors of metabolites in the system.

Beyond relationships between metabolites, metabolic systems can be analysed under the polymorphism concept consisting in identifying different metabolic poles or trends representing output products or responses of system. Such identification can be achieved by correspondence analysis which extracts the extreme metabolic profiles showing the highest regulations for some metabolites. By reference to these metabolic trends, all the metabolic profiles of the population can be classified into homogeneous groups by means of cluster analysis. At population level, the metabolic profiles represent polymorphic units of the metabolic system.

Beyond correlations between metabolites and associations of metabolic profiles to metabolic trends, a third variability can be analysed consisting of atypical profiles in the population due to atypical values for some metabolites. Identification of such atypical cases can be achieved by means of different outlier diagnostics. Outlier extraction leads to homogenize the studied population on the hand, and can bring interesting information on eventual new populations on the other hand.

A part from static analysis, metabolic systems can be analysed under kinetic or dynamic aspects by considering the variations of parameters (e.g. concentrations) in time. Time-dependent variation analysis includes deterministic compartment models, stochastic fitting and dynamic stability analysis.

These different computational approaches to variability analysis of metabolic systems are presented in this book and illustrated by different numerical applications and figures.

DEDICATION

To my Professor, Maurice ROUX

(Aix-Marseille 3, Marseilles, France)

INTRODUCTION

Metabolic systems are characterized by a high variability in chemical structures, biosynthesis levels, regulation ratios and flux distributions of metabolites (Kacser and Burns, 1973; Savageau, 1976; Atkinson, 1977; Hayashi and Sakamoto, 1986; Fell, 1996; Heinrich and Schuster, 1996). Such variability is controlled by different processes and governing factors which manifest at different structural and functional levels. These levels extend from metabolites to metabolic profiles via metabolic reactions and metabolic pathways.

Concerning the processes responsible for the metabolic variability, they can be intrinsic or extrinsic to metabolic system: intrinsic processes include flux distributions, enzymatic regulations and competitions; also, metabolic systems are organized into different pathways which represent a key topological factor controlling the functionality and evolution of such systems. Extrinsic factors include genetic regulations, physiological states and environmental conditions which can significantly stimulate, modulate or repress the metabolism.

Metabolomics aims at unbiased and comprehensive analysis of the biosynthesis, regulation, distribution and control processes of the metabolites in cells, tissues or organisms (Figure 1) (Goodacre et al., 2004; Sumner et al., 2003; Kell, 2004; Sweetlove and Fernie, 2005; Fernie et al., 2004). It is a multidisciplinary field including many approaches to analyse the metabolic content and variability of a biological system in relation to several biotic and abiotic factors (genome, proteome, physiology, environment). Subsequent results will usefully help to understand more the organizations and behaviors of metabolic networks (Olivier et al., 1998; Roessner et el., 2001; Nicholson et al., 1999; Kell, 2002; Ott et al., 2003; Weckwerth, 2003).

Computational metabolomics aims at quantification and modeling of metabolic variability to gain more information on topological, functional and evolutive aspects of metabolism. For that, different computational methods can be applied to extract such information on different metabolic components including metabolites, metabolic (chemical) reactions, metabolic pathways and metabolic profiles (Figure 1) (Steuer, 2007).

(a)   **Different organisations of metabolic pathways (inside topology)**

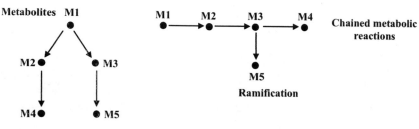

(b)   **Different regulation profiles of metabolites (outside typology)**

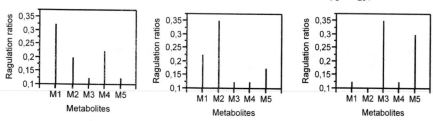

(c)   **Different metabolic control processes (functionality)**

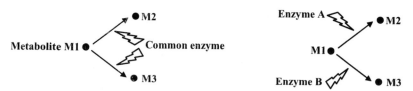

Figure 1. Schematic representations of different objectives in metabolomics. Analysis of pathways' organization (a), phenotypic expressions (b) and control processes (c) of metabolic networks.

At metabolite level, correlation analysis can be applied to quantify relationships (links) between the different chemical compounds of system. These relationships include affinities and oppositions between metabolites, and can be quantified by means of correlation coefficients (Steuer, 2006; Camacho et al., 2005). Positive and negative correlations can be generally interpreted in terms of shared or disputed factors between metabolites, respectively. Such preliminary information helps to be more familiar with the global organization and some functional aspects of the metabolic system. For wide metabolomic datasets containing many metabolites, correlation analysis can be applied by multivariate methods such as the principle component analysis (PCA). Also, correlation analysis includes sensitivity analysis of metabolism toward intrinsic or extrinsic control factors. Such approach is known by metabolic control analysis (MCA) (Kacser and Burns, 1973; Morgan and Rhodes, 2002; Castrillo et al., 2007).

Preliminary relationships highlighted by correlation analysis can be mathematically formalized (in a next step) by means of different modeling techniques. Such techniques include linear regression which can be applied on measured, transformed or latent variables. Transformations are needed when measured variables are not normally distributed. Latent variables are "synthetic" variables condensing information of several other (measured) ones. They are used in complex situations containing great numbers of (heterogeneous) variables.

At a higher level than metabolites, chemical reactions can be considered to apply stoichiometric analysis of metabolic system (Llaneras and Picó, 2008; Provost and Bastin, 2004; Calik and Ozdamar, 2002). Information on the chemical reactions will be numerically translated into a stoichiometric matrix of the system (topological information) and a vector of intracellular (unknown) and extracellular input-output (known) fluxes. Such information are combined to determine algebraically the intracellular fluxes representing the internal functional state of the metabolic system.

Beyond single reactions, topological analysis of metabolic networks can be deepened by computational identification of metabolic pathways. These components consist of independent serial of chemical reactions linking initial substrates to final products (Figure 1a) (Klamt and Stelling, 2003; Papin et al., 2003, 2004; Schuster and Hilgetag, 1994; Trinh et al., 2009). Such approach includes elementary mode and extreme pathway analyses (EMA and EPA).

Beyond the topological aspects, chemical reactions and metabolic pathways can be analyzed under a functional aspect by optimizing their properties or their output products (fluxes, concentrations, growths, etc.) in relation to well defined governing factors or constraints. Such analysis is known by flux balance analysis (FBA) (Lee et al., 2006).

Apart from the topological and functional analyses of metabolic networks (referring to metabolic maps), typological analyses can be performed to identify variability poles or metabolic trends from the whole variability contained in a set of metabolic profiles of the studied population. At population level, metabolic profiles are considered as basic components containing rich information on chemical responses and polymorphisms (Figure 1b): by definition, typological analysis aims at the search of different "types" into a population that will help to understand the complex diversity (polymorphism) of such a population. It can be carried out by means of cluster analysis (ClA) consisting in classifying the metabolic profiles into homogeneous groups based on similarity criteria (Everitt et al., 2001; Gordon, 1999; Roux, 1991a, b; Semmar et al., 2005).

Moreover, at population level, the chemical polymorphism issued from the metabolic system is achieved by identifying extreme metabolic trends associating high regulations of some metabolites to some metabolic profiles. This can be achieved by means of correspondence analysis (CA) (Greenacre, 1984, 1993; Escofier and Pages, 1991).

At the limit of population level, correlation and typological analyses can be combined to screen the presence of outliers. Outliers are atypical or extreme cases that can be identified on the basis of their distance calculations with respect to reference or typical profiles representative of the whole population (Filzmoser et al., 2005; Rousseeuw and Leroy, 1987; Barnett and Lewis, 1994; Andrews, 1972; Everitt and Dunn, 1992; Mortier and Bar-Hen, 2004; Swaroop and Winter, 1971; Robinson, 2005). Such outliers can be indicative of some exceptional cases, experimental errors, extreme evolutionary trends or new populations.

Functional links between metabolic levels regulations (by the central machine) and the output metabolic profiles can be statistically explored by combining the variabilities within and between profiles belonging to different metabolic trends. This can be achieved by applying the weighted metabolic profile analysis (WMPA) (Semmar, 2010).

Beyond the static aspect, kinetic and dynamic analyses can be applied to fit or to predict variations of concentrations or fluxes in time. For a given metabolite, predictive kinetic models of concentration can be established by either deterministic or stochastic approaches: deterministic models give directly the concentration levels in the system at any time, whereas stochastic models are based on probability laws from which the total concentration in the system will be reduced to punctual levels along time (considered as random variable) (Bonate, 2006; Heikkilä, 1999; Matis and Wehrly, 1990; Wimmer et al., 1999; Lansky, 1996).

Deterministic approach will be illustrated in this book by compartment modeling based on the decomposition of concentration-time curves into different "homogeneous" variation phases (Bonate, 2006; Holz and Fahr, 2001; Ritschel and Kearns, 1999).

Stochastic approach will be illustrated in this book by the Weibull law which is advantageously flexible to fit different shapes of kinetic curves (Heikkilä, 1999).

Beyond single variable cases (e.g. concentrations of one metabolite), dynamic analysis can be performed to explore the behavior of metabolic system with respect to several variables (e.g. concentrations of several metabolites). Such analysis can be achieved by means of a theoretical approach based on partial derivatives of velocity function with respect to all the variables of system. The set of all the partial derivatives are then calculated at the equilibrium point giving the Jacobian matrix. Finally, the behavior of the system towards small perturbations can be deduced from the eigenvalues of the Jacobian matrix (Abraham and Shaw, 1981; Sprott, 2003, Strogatz, 2000; Steuer, 2007).

These different computational approaches applied to metabolomics are illustrated by several intuitive figures and by using numerical applications. Moreover, interpretations of results issued from numerical applications are presented by referring to different metabolic concepts and processes.

Chapter 1

MULTIPLE CLASSIFICATION OF METABOLOMIC APPROACHES

I. GENERAL LINES ON METABOLOMIC APPROACHES

Metabolomic approaches cover a wide library of computational tools that can be used to analyse metabolic systems under several aspects (Chou and Voit, 2009; Ishii et al., 2004; Goodacre et al., 2004; Crampin et al., 2004; Mrabet and Semmar, 2010). Such aspects can be classified by reference to four directive lines (Figure 1.1):

- Initial or basic information including data types and matrices representing the metabolic system (Figure 1.1a),
- Computational tools implying different types of results (Figure 1.1b),
- Methodological rules including different assumptions, conditions and constraints (if needed) required to solve metabolomic problems (Figure 1.1c).
- Working scale linked to the elementary components used to description of metabolic system (Figure 1.1d).

II. METABOLOMIC DATASETS AND MATRICIAL REPRESENTATIONS OF METABOLIC SYSTEMS

Initially, basic information describing metabolic systems can be static or time-dependent: a dataset of metabolites' concentrations in different individuals provides static information on the system. However, if different concentrations of a given metabolite are measured in different individuals at different times, the metabolic dataset acquires a kinetic aspect which requires kinetic approaches (Figure 1.2) (Steuer, 2007; Stelling, 2004; Varma and Palsson, 1994).

Apart from the measured static or kinetic data, complex information on metabolic systems (topologies, processes, evolutions) can be condensed and organized into different basic matrices, viz., connectivity (1), stoichiometric (2), transition probabilities (3), partial derivatives (4), mixed components (5) matrices , etc. (Rodriguez and Infante, 2009; Mrabet and Semmar, 2010; Durot et al., 2009; Chou and Voit, 2009; Baths et al., 2009; Malarz and Kułakowski, 2005) (Figure 1.1a).

II.1. Presentation of Metabolomic Datasets

A metabolomic dataset consists of several individuals (patients/animals/plants/cell cultures) in whom/which the concentrations of several metabolites were measured. The set of concentrations of p metabolites analysed in n individuals is stored into a matrix (n rows $\times$ p columns) (Figure 1.2). Each row of the concentration dataset represents initially a concentration profile and can be converted into a metabolic regulation ratio profile by dividing the concentration C_j of each metabolite j by the sum of concentrations of all the metabolites (Figure 1.3).

A metabolomic dataset can be static or kinetic whether its n rows are measured at a single time or at different times (Figure 1.2). In the second case, the concentrations of a given metabolite j measured at different times in a same individual i gives the kinetic profile of such a metabolite in such an individual. Therefore, the n concentration values of a given metabolite can be organized into q ($q < n$) kinetic profiles containing successive concentrations observed in the q studied individuals (e.g. q patients).

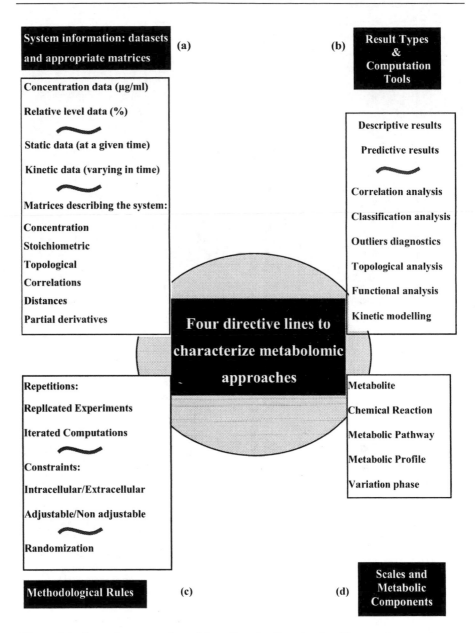

Figure 1.1. General presentation of four directive lines to classify or to characterize metabolomic approaches.

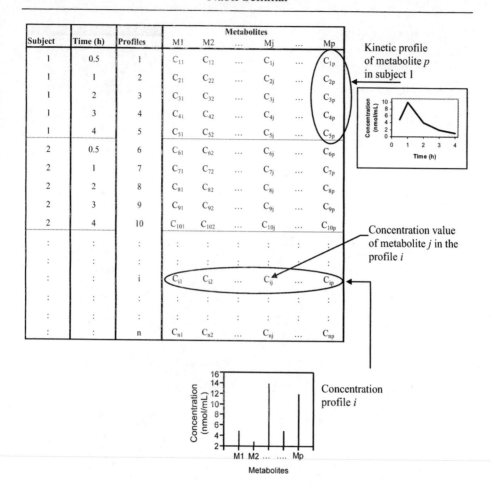

Figure 1.2. Representation of a metabolomic dataset (n profiles $\times$ p metabolites) with its different parameters. Concentration (static) and kinetic profiles are read along rows and columns, respectively.

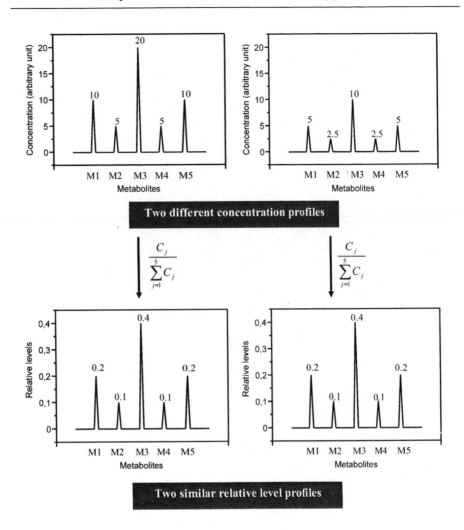

Figure 1.3. Standardization of concentration profiles giving relative level (or regulation) profiles.

II.2. Static versus Kinetic Approaches

Static and kinetic (or dynamic) approaches refer to analysis of system using data or formulations in which time is neglected and considered, respectively. In the first case (static), a dataset is initially treated as a whole block which will be mathematically decomposed into topological or functional components or states characterizing the system. In the second case (kinetic), a dataset is initially undertaken as succession of different phases varying in time leading to successive pictures representing sequential behaviors of the system (Figure 1.4).

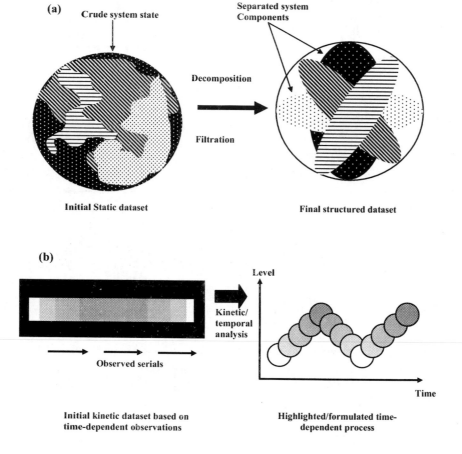

Figure 1.4. Intuitive representations of static (a) and kinetic/temporal (b) analyses.

Static approaches include:

- Topological analysis of metabolic maps (Janga and Babu, 2008; Yetukuri et al., 2007).

- Flux distribution analysis through metabolic networks (Blank and Kuepfer, 2010; Ishii et al., 2004; Williams et al., 2008; Sriram et al., 2004; Kruger et al., 2003).
- Correlation analysis between metabolites' levels and their associations to different intracellular and extracellular factors (Steuer, 2006; Camacho et al., 2005).
- Chemical polymorphism analysis through the classification of metabolic profiles into homogeneous clusters representing different metabolic trends (MbTrs) which are characterized by different regulation ratios (Semmar, 2010).

Kinetic or dynamic approaches include:

- Analysis of variation phases in concentration-time curves from which (i) kinetic parameters can be directly calculated, and (ii) fitting models of concentration in time can be developed (Bonate, 2006; Semmar and Simon, 2006).
- Deterministic modeling of time-dependent concentrations based on differential equations set (Yugi et al., 2005).
- Dynamical stability analysis of a system based on its theoretical perturbation at initial time, followed by its ability or no to return to equilibrium according to one or several possible ways. For that, Jacobian matrix needs to be calculated (Tuljapurkar and Caswell, 1997; Yang et al., 2004).
- Modeling of metabolic system evolution based on enzymatic kinetics (Michaelis-Menten kinetics) (Piazza et al., 2008; Ralser et al., 2007; Wu et al., 2005; Crampin et al., 2004; Campbell, 1990; Ralser et al., 2007).
- Stochastic (probabilistic) modeling of concentration-time variability based on continuous time Markov chains with finite number of states (Aronson and Kellog, 1978; Matis, 1988).
- Stochastic analysis of retention or residence time of metabolite particles in metabolic system based on the use/determination of appropriate probability density functions (Matis, 1988; Chiang, 1980; Matis and Wehrly, 1990; Semmar and Simon, 2006).

II.3. Matricial Representations and Formulations of Metabolic Systems

Metabolic systems are known to be complex networks in which many components/processes are interconnected. Representations of such inter-connections and the encoding of functional processes require matrix formulations which represent flexible tools to store multi-path information. On this basis, different metabolomic approaches can be considered by reference to the matrix tool used for metabolic system analysis. Matrix tools can be used to describe/compute distances, correlations, connectivities, transition probabilities, transformation reactions, equilibrium and mixture states between different components of biological (metabolic) system (Figures 1.7-1.10) (Crampin et al., 2004; Semmar et al., 2001, 2005b, 2008 ; Sumner et al., 2003; Gonzalez-Diaz et al., 2008; Gonzalez-Diaz, 2008; Kose et al., 2001; Llaneras and Picó, 2008; Steuer, 2007; Stelling, 2004).

Correlation matrix gives correlation coefficients between all the metabolites' pairwises (or other variables of system) (Figure 1.5). Such coefficients are calculated from experimental data (e.g. concentration of metabolites), and can be positive or negative with absolute values varying between 0 and 1. An absolute value close to 1 can be indicative of a strong relationship between metabolites. Positive correlations reveal functional affinities between metabolites, whereas negative correlations indicate functional oppositions between metabolites. Such affinities and oppositions are linked to the topology of metabolic map, the sensitivities of metabolites toward some control parameters and the distributions of enzymatic activities within the network system. Interpretations of correlations between metabolites will be detailed in chapter 3 (§II.4).

Distance matrix quantifies similarities and dissimilarities between all the individuals (e.g. metabolic profiles) of studied population (e.g. metabolic system). The distances between metabolic profiles are calculated taking into account the differences between levels of all theirs respective metabolites (Figure 1.6).

Neighbouring states or links between all the metabolites in a metabolic map can be encoded by using Bolean connectivity matrix. Connectivity between such components is encoded by using a binary formalism (Boolean code) consisting of 1 if two components (metabolites) are connected and 0 if not (Estrada and Bodin, 2008; Estrada, 2006, 2007; Vilar et al., 2005; Kose et al., 2001; Janga and Babu, 2008). For instance, the value 1 can be attributed for two metabolites which are spatially neighbour (e.g. belonging to a same metabolic pathway) or which are directly linked (e.g. precursor-product) (Figure 1.7). The resulting adjacency matrix can be graphically represented by a multigraph containing p nodes or vertices (corresponding to the p components) which are connected by edges.

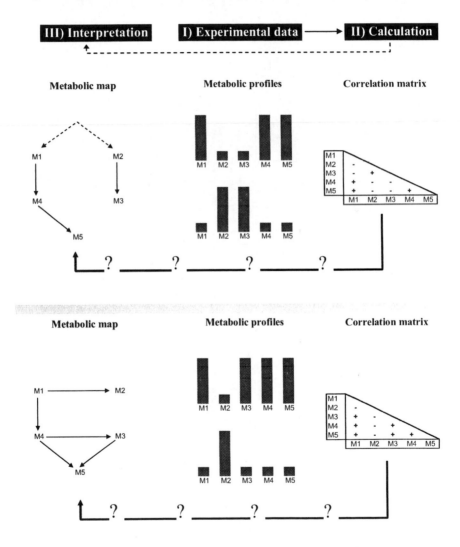

Figure 1.5. Two examples illustrating topological interpretations of metabolic maps from correlation matrices calculated from different experimental metabolic profiles.

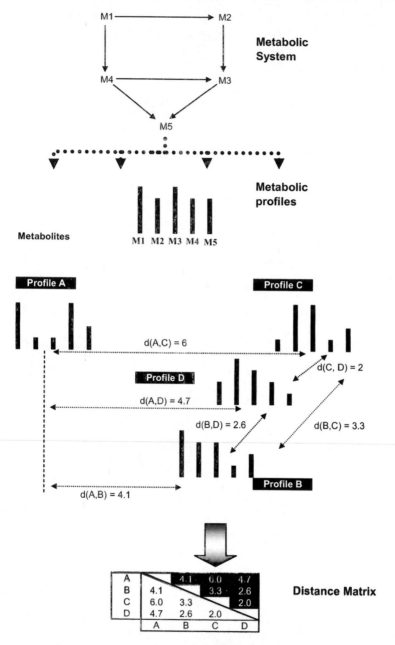

Figure 1.6. Intuitive illustration on distance matrix calculation between five metabolic profiles quantifying similarities/dissimilarities between them.

Metabolites	Unchanged states	Transformation reactions	
M1	M1 → M1	M1 → M2	M1 → M4
M2	M2 → M2	M2 → M3	M2 → M4
M3	M3 → M3	M3 → M4	M3 → M5
M4	M4 → M4	M4 → M5	
M5	M5 → M5		

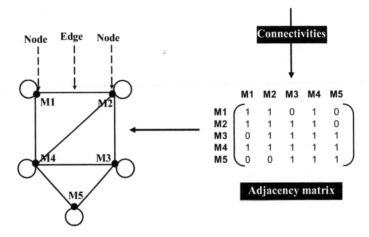

Figure 1.7. Boolean formalism of connectivities between metabolites in a metabolic system and corresponding graphical representation.

Transition probabilities matrix gives the probabilities of each metabolite to be transformed into another or more generally to transit from a state to another. This leads to a finite number of successive states (Guttorp, 1995; Tamir, 1998). The transition concept can be generalized to any variation in the state of a biological (metabolic) system in time. For example, at a given time, a metabolic system can be described by the set of the metabolites present in the network. Between two successive times t and $t+1$, each molecule of metabolite j can be subjected to different mutually exclusive processes: it can remain unchanged, or be transformed to another metabolite among other possible ones. The exclusivity between the different metabolic processes makes possible to analyse the evolution of the metabolic system on the basis of transition probabilities of metabolites through different successive states. These probabilities ($0 \leq\, \leq 1$) are stored into a transition matrix the rows and columns of which represent the initial (e.g. precursor) and final (e.g. product) elements (Figure 1.8). For a given metabolite (a component of the system), the sum of all transition probabilities is equal to 1.

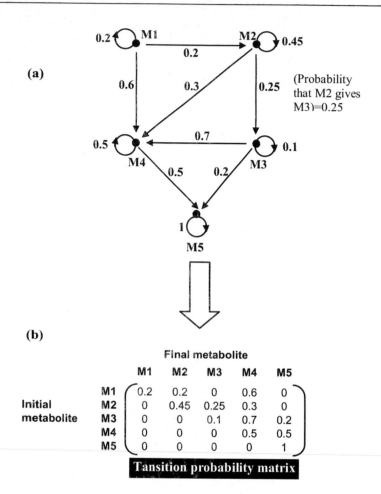

Figure 1.8. Basic example representing a transition probability matrix (b) and its graphical representation (a).

Stoichiometric matrix gives the stoichiometric coefficients of each metabolite in the different chemical reactions of metabolic system. Metabolites and reactions represent the rows and columns of stoichiometric matrix, respectively (Figure 1.9). A stoichiometric coefficient represents the number of molecules of a given metabolite consumed or produced by a given elementary reaction. Stoichiometric coefficients take positive or negative values for appearing (products) and disappearing (reactants) metabolites, respectively. At the scale of whole metabolic system, such algebraic coefficients are balanced between them, i.e. between products and reactants.

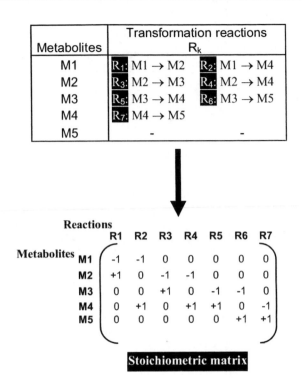

Figure 1.9. Representation of all the chemical reactions in a metabolic network by a stoichiometric matrix containing the stoichiometric coefficients, i.e. the numbers of molecules of different metabolites appearing and disappearing from these reactions.

When different components of a system are implied in a same final response, they can be mathematically undertaken under linear combination concept. Linear combinations can be used to represent different types of mixtures in which the different components have different weights or contributions. Statistically, the weights of q components implied in different mixture states of the system are given by Scheffé's mixture matrix. In other words, this matrix shows how the relative parts (contributions, weights) of different components vary to give different final mixture products characterizing the system capability. The total number of mixtures in Schéffé's matrix can be calculated from the number (q) of components to mix and the maximum number of mixture levels (m) for each component. An illustration of a Schéffé's matrix for $q=3$ and $m=5$ is given in Figure 1.10. More details on mixture design based on Scheffé's matrix will be presented in chapter 6.

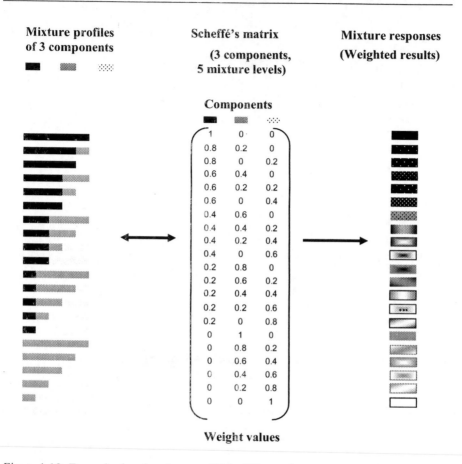

| Mixture profiles of 3 components | Scheffé's matrix (3 components, 5 mixture levels) | Mixture responses (Weighted results) |

Weight values

Figure 1.10. Example showing the use of Scheffé's matrix to encode a complete set of mixtures between different (three) components leading to different mixture responses.

Dynamic behaviors of different system components, the ones with respect to the others, can be analysed by using partial derivatives. Dynamic behaviors are associated to a perturbed system the new equilibrium of which can be reached or no according to different ways. A simplistic example on dynamic stability is given by pendulum system (Figure 1.11a). Initially, the parameters or components x_j need to be expressed as analytical functions of time, i.e. $x_j(t)$. Then, the dynamical behavior of perturbed system to return to or to diverge from equilibrium can be analysed from its Jacobian matrix J (Figure 1.11). This matrix gives the partial derivative values (df_j/dx_j) of flow functions f_j characterizing the multivariate behavior of system with reference to all its time-dependent parameters $x_j(t)$. Then, the partial derivatives will be calculated at equilibrium point, i.e. where the variations of the parameters $x_j(t)$

in time are null ($dx_j/dt=0$) (Figure 1.11). Finally, the system behavior will be directly interpreted from the calculated eigenvalues of J.

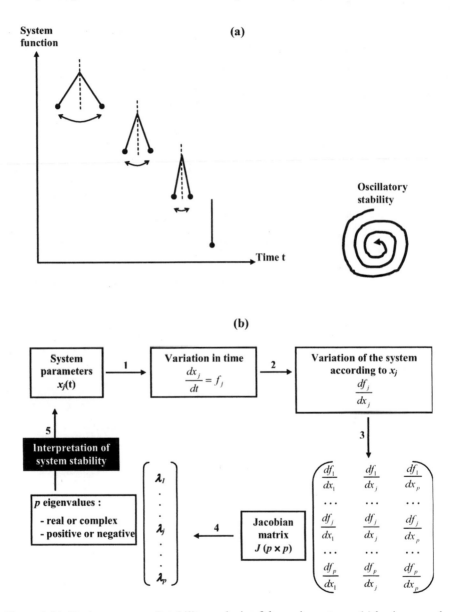

Figure 1.11. Basic concepts of stability analysis of dynamic systems; (a) basic example of a dynamic stability; (b) establishment and usefulness of Jacobian matrix to stability analysis of dynamic system.

III. CLASSIFICATION OF METABOLOMIC APPROACHES ACCORDING TO COMPUTATIONAL TOOLS AND RESULT TYPES

III.1. Descriptive versus Predictive Approaches

Metabolomic approaches can be classified according to two methodological aspects giving two types of results: one can distinguish descriptive and predictive approaches which are applied to describe and to predict complex structures/behaviors of metabolic systems, respectively (Figures 1.12; 1.1b).

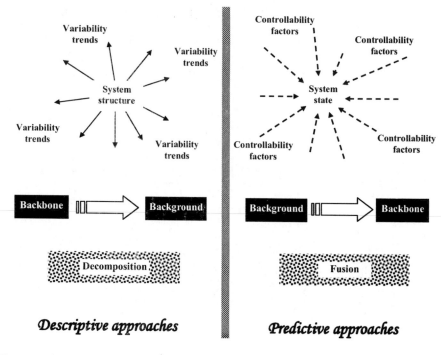

Figure 1.12. Schematic representation of the general goals in descriptive and predictive approaches.

Descriptive approaches consider initially the system as a whole block (backbone) from which different variability trends or components (background) are generated by appropriate decomposition techniques. Thus, the whole system will be decomposed to highlight different components

(Figure 1.12): metabolic systems have network structures characterized by multidimensional organizations and multivariate functionalities. Such a complexity needs to be simplified by decomposing it into different components helping to understand more the structures and behaviors of the whole complex system. In summary, decomposition concept represents a strong methodological basis to describe the complex structures and to highlight different variability trends in metabolic (biological) systems.

Descriptive approaches include topological, correlation and classification analyses applied of different system components (Figure 1.1.b):

I.   Topological analysis aims at identification of the whole system organization through analysis of interaction and connection between its components (metabolites, reactions, pathways).

II.   Correlation analysis aims at quantification of links between variables (e.g. metabolites' concentrations) of metabolic system. According to their oppositions or affinities, the variables will be associated to common or different metabolic trends (Semmar et al.,2001; Fendt et al., 2010; Weckwerth and Morgental, 2005).

III. Classification analysis is based on distance computations between metabolic profiles; this helps to highlight chemical polymorphisms in biological populations leading to understand the typology generated by the metabolic system.

IV.   By combining correlation and classification analyses, another aspect of descriptive approaches can be applied consisting in identifying atypical cases or outliers in the studied population.

Predictive approaches aim to predict the behavior of the system subjected to different variation or controllability factors. The general methodological aspect (aim, steps) is inverted compared to that of descriptive approaches: different variability factors are combined to estimate precisely what internal state could be reached by the system (Figure 1.12). This helps to identify the most significant factors which control the system.

In metabolomics, predictive approaches include different modeling techniques helping to fit concentration or flux variations in time or in relation to control parameter(s) (Figure 1.1.b) (Antoniewicz et al., 2006; Kotte et al., 2010; Steuer et al., 2006; Smallbone et al., 2007; Piazza et al., 2008).

III.2. COMPUTATIONAL TOOLS ASSOCIATED TO DESCRIPTIVE APPROACHES

Descriptive approaches include several computational tools which are appropriate to analyse the complexity of metabolic systems under different decomposition concepts:

Network topology analysis, based on graph theory, is used to characterize the complex network structure of a metabolic map by decomposing it into nodes (metabolites) connected by edges (neighboring links or transformation reactions) (Figure 1.7) (Rodriguez and Infante, 2009; Steuer, 2007). From the adjacency matrix representing the connectivities between metabolites, several indicator coefficients can be calculated to characterize and to interpret the network structure.

Stoichiometric analysis describes a metabolic system on the basis of elementary chemical reactions linking the different metabolites (substrates and products) of the system (Llaneras and Picó, 2008; Poolman et al., 2004). It includes different approaches among which metabolic pathway analysis is applied to describe a metabolic system by a minimal number of functional units, the metabolic pathways. Such pathways are defined as independent serial of chemical reactions connecting initial substrates to final products (Figure 2.7) (Trinh et al., 2009; Price et al., 2004; Papin et al., 2003). They represent high-scale topological and functional components in the metabolic systems.

The variability of a metabolomic dataset containing n profiles and p metabolites (n rows $\times$ p columns) can be analyzed by different descriptive techniques based on distance and/or correlation calculations. Three types of analyses can be applied, viz. along rows, along columns, and by associating rows and columns (Figure 1.13) (Lindon et al. 2007; Sumner et al., 2003):

Column analysis organizes the metabolic system into metabolites varying the ones with respect to the others. It focuses on the relationships between such variables (metabolites) by calculating correlation coefficients between them (Steuer, 2006; Camacho et al., 2005). In the case of large datasets containing great numbers of columns (and rows), affinities and oppositions between the numerous metabolites can be explored by means of principle component analysis, a multivariate technique decomposing a dataset into eigenvalues and eigenvectors (Wishart, 2007).

Row analysis organizes the metabolic system into subsets of metabolic profiles which will be grouped or separated according to their sharing degrees of the whole variability. Similarities and differences between such profiles are analysed through distance or similarity coefficient calculations. This helps to classify the individuals into homogeneous groups that can be interpreted as polymorphism poles of the studied population. Such a fine segmentation of the dataset (population) can be reliably performed by means of cluster analysis (Semmar et al., 2005b; Everitt et al., 2001; Gordon, 1999; Arabie et al., 1996).

By considering both the rows (profiles) and columns (metabolites), extreme, atypical or original associations between some individual profiles and variables can be identified in the dataset (Figure 1.14). Such a heterogeneity or diversity analysis can be performed by means of different outlier diagnostics (Chapter 5).

Finally, it is worthy to note that the well structured results given by descriptive approaches provide meticulous information that can be used to improve the results of predictive approaches.

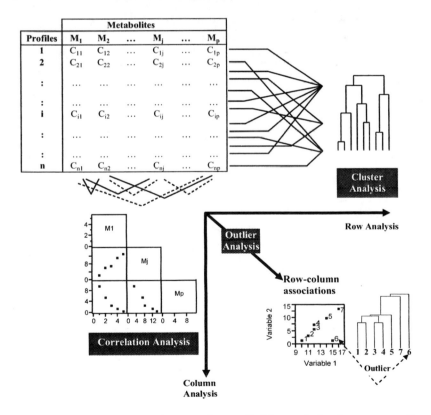

Figure 1.13. Different statistical approaches applied in metabolomics corresponding to horizontal or vertical data analysis.

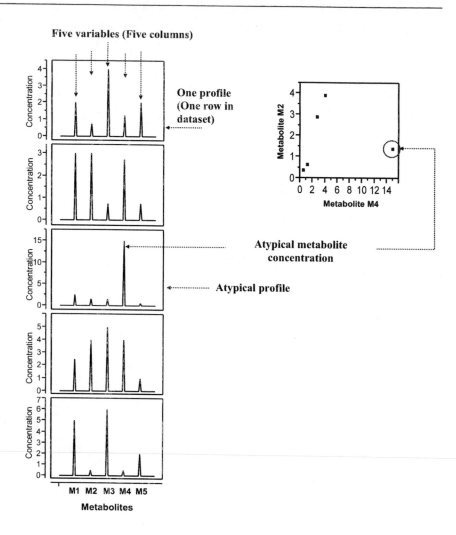

Figure 1.14. Simple illustration of identification of atypical profile(s) and associated concentration value(s) based on profile (row) and variable (column) analyses, respectively.

III.3. COMPUTATIONAL TOOLS ASSOCIATED TO PREDICTIVE APPROACHES

Predictive approaches include several tools which can be applied to different metabolic questions:

- Prediction of metabolites' concentrations in a biological matrix (compartment) in relation to different time-varying processes including absorption, biosynthesis, distribution, storage, transformation and elimination. Such approaches are commonly applied in pharmacokinetic modeling (Bonate, 2006; Welling, 1997; Boroujerdi, 2002; Shargel and Yu, 1999).
- Prediction of metabolites' concentrations and their regulation levels in metabolic systems in relation to presence/absence, type and concentration of single enzymes on the hand, and interactions between enzymes on the other hand (Piazza et al., 2008).
- Prediction of metabolic responses in relation to internal characteristics (genetics, physiology, etc.) of biological system or to external factors (e.g. temperature, pH, etc.) (Lewis et al., 2008). Such questions can be solved by means of flux balance analysis (Resendis-Antonio, 2007). Also, responses of biological populations to drugs are modeled by means of different pharmacodynamic methods (Bonate, 2006).

IV. DIFFERENT METHODOLOGICAL RULES FOR METABOLOMIC APPROACHES

Analysis of metabolic systems needs different methodological rules to overcome some unavoidable difficulties with complex and highly variable systems. Such difficulties can be summarized by the following points:

- Complex topological organization of metabolic network
- High dimension variability space
- High number of factors governing the system
- High number of internal states resulting from high variability of system parameters
- Imparity in variance or variation magnitude of different components
- Permanent variations leading to dynamical and probabilistic aspects of the system.

These difficulties can be overcame by different methodological rules leading to simplification, filtration, homogenization, categorization and reliability of information concerning the studied complex system. Such rules include:

- Repeatability to surround the average behavior (characteristics) of system (Steuer, 2006; Semmar, 2010).
- Random sampling to take care neutrality in information collection from large biological populations leading to unbiased results on corresponding systems (Legendre and Legendre, 2000; Semmar, 2010).
- Homogenization of variability scales through data standardization (transformation). Data transformations include also a great number of techniques which are appropriately applied to guarantee linearity and normality (Veflingstad et al., 2004; Smallbone et al., 2007).
- Decomposition of the system into different components to access its organizational and functional structures (Mrabet and Semmar, 2010; Antoniewicz et al., 2006; Fendt et al., 2010; Wishart, 2007; Wienkoop et al., 2008).
- Imposition of constraints to the system to limit (to control) its high variability filed (Llaneras and Pico, 2008; Stelling, 2004).

IV.1. Repeated Measurement Requirement

The variability in biological systems is complex because of a high number of non-controllable factors leading to a random character of such systems. Perpetual fluctuations of the systems under such factors generate a probabilistic behavior which can be overcame by searching the most frequent (average) state of the system among all the possible ones. For that, repeated measurements (or replicates) are needed to gain information on the variability and the most probable (average) state of the system (Figure 1.15). Such repetitions will help to localize the position of the central state of system as well as the variation range around such a state.

Single measurements are not sufficient to extract reliable information on system backbone, and even under approximately constant experimental conditions, metabolism is a highly dynamic/sensitive system, responding to small factor (stimuli) variations. For example, slight differences in enzyme concentrations or metabolic fluxes (among other factors) contribute to significant variations in metabolite levels. The results are metabolic fluctuations which propagate through metabolic reaction chains and ultimately induce different patterns of metabolites (Steuer et al., 2003a, b; Weckwerth, 2003; Weckwerth et al., 2004 a, b; Morgenthal et al., 2005, 2006). Variability between and within such patterns can be statistically surrounded through replicated chemical analyses.

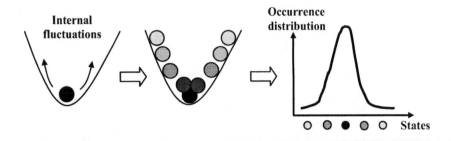

Figure 1.15. Internal fluctuations of a system resulting in a characteristic distribution of its different possible states. Therefore, reliable analysis requires replicated measurements to surround the central (most stable) position, variation range and distribution of the states of system.

IV.2. Randomisation or Random Sampling

Randomisation is a general rule in population analysis which avoids the bias of selected results leading to under-estimation of the system (population) variability. It consists in randomly sampling individuals (elements or components) in the studied infinite population to obtain a finite number of samples representative of such a population. The population can be sampled as a whole block or after its stratification into homogeneous parts, but in all the cases, the individuals must be collected by the rule of simple random sampling. For that, random numbers table can be used to affect numbers to all the individuals of the population, then to collect the n first individuals corresponding to the n first decreasing (or increasing) random numbers.

IV.3. Data Standardization

Data standardization is required when the variables of system have different units or different variances. Its gives dimensionless variables with unit standard deviation leading to express all the values of dataset on a common standard scale.

Standardization is fundamental in correlation analysis. Also, it provides appropriate results for comparisons between different systems or different states of a same system.

In the case where variables have the same unit, standardization can be applied to avoid that variables with high variances dominate those with low variances.

IV.4. Constraint Requirement

Metabolism is characterized by a great number of states originating from numerous interactive components and resulting in high variability and multidimensional behavior of the system. Analyses of the high variability and multidimensionality of a metabolic system are limited by the fact that some components and states (especially intracellular) are not accessible experimentally. To overcome such problems, some constraints or assumptions on state, functionality or capacity of the system are needed. From such constraints, the variability space of the complex system will be delimited to be well defined geometrically (Figure 1.16). Subsequently to constraints definitions, different processes governing the system will be identified and controlled.

The different constraints can be classified according to different ways, viz. intracellular or extracellular (I, II), and non adjustable or adjustable (III, IV) (Figure 1.17):

I.   Intracellular constraints include steady state, flux irreversibility, flux capacity. These constraints are at the basis of mathematical equations and inequalities giving solutions on states, regulatory processes and optimal behaviors of metabolic systems.
II.   Extracellular constraints include substrate uptakes/limitations, environmental conditions (temperature, pH, light, etc.) as well as interactions between biological systems.
III.   Non adjustable constraints imply time-invariant restrictions to possible cell behaviors including those linked to thermodynamics (e.g. irreversibility of fluxes), stoichiometry (e.g. steady state balance) and enzyme or transport capacities (e.g. maximum flux values) (Figure 1.18).
IV.   Adjustable constraints depend on environmental conditions or experimental designs; they may change through time and vary

between individuals (cells, organisms, populations) by opposition to the non-adjustable constraints. Enzyme kinetics, genetic modifications and planned experimental conditions provide examples of adjustable constraints (Llaneras and Picó, 2007, 2008; Edwards et al., 2002). By opposition to the invariant (non-adjustable) constraints which are always satisfied, the results issued from adjustable constraints are valid only under the considered experimental circumstances.

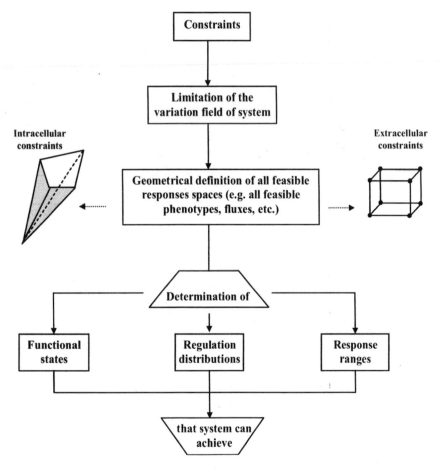

Figure 1.16. Requirement of constraints to extract properties of complex systems through the delimiation of their high variability spaces.

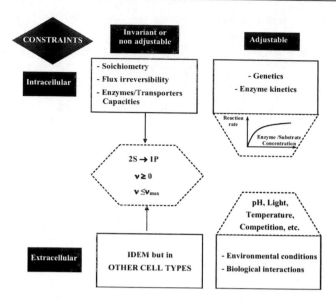

Figure 1.17. Classification of different constraints used in different metabolomic approaches to overcome multidimensionality, high variability and limited accessibility of metabolic systems. Legend: S, substrate; P, product; ν, reaction flux.

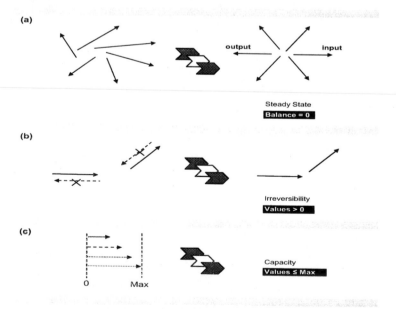

Figure 1.18. Illustrations of different time-invariant (non-adjustable) constraints that can be applied to analyse metabolic systems.

V. METABOLOMIC APPROACHES
LINKED TO DECOMPOSITION
SCALES OF METABOLIC SYSTEMS

V.1. Metabolic Components

Metabolic systems can be undertaken at different scales corresponding to different units or components (Figure 1.19) (Mrabet and Semmar, 2010; Jamshidi and Palsson, 2008). Such components vary from metabolites (i) to metabolic profiles (iv) via chemical reactions (ii) and metabolic pathways (iii). They give to metabolic systems structural (i), elementary functional (ii), global regulatory (iii) and output polymorphic (iv) aspects. Metabolic profiles (iv) condense information and variability of the three other components (i, ii, iii) to give a high-scale picture on the chemical variability in biological populations. They are appropriate parameters to highlight flexibility and evolutive trends of metabolism in such populations (Semmar, 2010).

System components can have a temporal dimension consisting of successive variation phases appearing in a time range. Such phases represent a basis in kinetic and dynamic analyses of metabolic systems (Chou and Voit, 2009; Mrabet and Semmar, 2010; Semmar and Simon, 2006).

V.2. Associations between Metabolomic
Approaches and Metabolic Components

The different metabolic components are analysed from different datasets by using different mathematical/statistical approaches (Figure 1.19):

A metabolic system can be simply (initially) considered as a set of different metabolites characterized by their concentrations. Under such decomposition, correlations between metabolites can be analysed by means of bivariate or multivariate techniques. Bivariate techniques consist in calculating correlation coefficients between metabolites pairwises. Such correlations can be parametric (e.g. Pearson's) or non-parametric (e.g. Spearman's)   (Zar, 1999; Camacho et al., 2005; Morgenthal et al., 2006; Semmar et al., 2001; Tikunov et al., 2005). Multivariate techniques provide factorial maps in which all the trends between metabolites can be represented at once leading to complete analysis of their relative affinities/oppositions. Such techniques include the principle component analysis (PCA) which helps to understand complex variabilities and structures of large metabolomic datasets (Guebel et al., 2009; Tiziani et al., 2009; Tikunov et al., 2005; Zhen et al., 2007).

By considering the metabolic systems as a set of chemical reactions between different metabolites, stoichiometric analyses can be applied to understand the organizational and functional states of the system: metabolic flux analysis (MFA) aims at determination how metabolic fluxes are distributed through all the intracellular chemical reactions (Llaneras and Picó, 2008; Ettenhuber et al., 2005; Kruger et al., 2003).

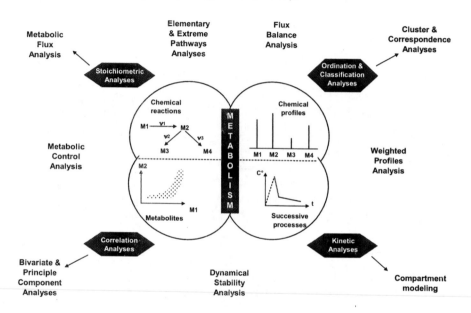

Figure 1.19. Classification of computational metabolomic approaches on the basis of different decomposition concepts of metabolic system. Legend: M1-M4, Metabolites M1-M4. v: flux. t, time. C°, concentration.

By considering the known stoichiometry of a metabolic system, one would like to determine fluxes giving an optimal biological response mathematically translated as an objective function (to maximize or to minimize) (e.g. ATP production, cell growth, etc.). This aim can be approached by means of flux balance analysis (FBA) (Motter et al., 2008; Edwards et al., 2002; Resendis-Antonio, 2007).

Metabolic control analysis (MCA), intermediate between correlation and stoichiometric analyses, aims at determination correlations between metabolic flux distributions and some governing factors including genetic and kinetic constraints (Kacser and Burns, 1973; Morgan and Rhodes, 2002; Castrillo et al., 2007; Yang et al., 1998; Wildermuth, 2000).

At a functional scale higher than chemical reaction, a metabolic system can be decomposed into different metabolic pathways representing independent functional units and consisting of serials of chemical reactions working according to autonomous ways. The identification of such metabolic pathways can be obtained by elementary mode analysis (EMA) (Schilling et al., 1999). Moreover, such functionally independent pathways (or elementary modes) can be restricted to a minimum number of mathematically independent pathways, called extreme pathways (EP), from which any functional pathway can be generated by an appropriate linear combination. The determination of EP is performed by extreme pathway analysis (EPA) (Price et al., 2004; Palsson et al., 2003).

Beyond the intracellular metabolic pathways, metabolic systems can be analysed from their output products consisting of metabolic profiles which represent high scale components. Metabolic profiles vary the ones from the others by different regulation ratios (relative levels) of metabolites. The variability contained in the set of all the metabolic profiles can be statistically analysed to highlight chemical polymorphism the origins of which can be linked to differential functional states of metabolic pathways in the metabolic system. The chemical polymorphism is statistically highlighted by cluster analysis (ClA) which classifies all the metabolic profiles into homogeneous groups representing metabolic trends (MbTrs) (Roux, 1991a, b; Everitt et al., 2001; Gordon, 1999). Moreover, the characteristics of such MbTrs (exclusive occurrences, production and regulation levels of some metabolites) can be revealed by means of correspondence analysis (CA) (Greenacre, 1984, 1993; Escofier and Pages, 1991).

The different MbTrs highlighted by ClA and CA represent frank metabolic states originated from gradual (relative) variations in activities of metabolic pathways the ones at expense of the others. Between MbTrs, there are continuums of intermediate states that can be easily observed from the variability of metabolic datasets. Thus, all the analysed metabolic profiles can be more or less associated to different MbTrs according to their similarity or dissimilarity levels. Mathematically, intermediate states can be generated from combinations of metabolic profiles representing different MbTrs; on this basis, it becomes interesting to analyse how the observed chemical polymorphism can be generated by gradual expressions of the different MbTrs. This helps to approach metabolic processes responsible for observed chemical polymorphisms. Such analysis of metabolic origins of chemical polymorphism based on gradual combination of MbTrs can be performed by means of weighted metabolic profiles analysis (WMPA).

Apart from the static aspect, a metabolic system can be analysed in time by decomposing it into successive variation phases. For a given metabolite, the kinetic variations can be analysed by compartment modeling where different variation phases are conceptually associated to different compartments (Holz and Fahr, 2001; Boroujerdi, 2002; Shargel and Yu, 1999; Ritschel and Keam, 1999). Alternatively to such a variation phases-based modelling, global shapes of kinetic curves can be fitted on the basis of appropriate probability laws known by shapes' flexibility; this approach is known by stochastic modelling.

Finally, by considering two or more metabolites (two or more variables) in the system, their simultaneous variations or the effect of the one on the other in time can be subjected to dynamic stability analysis or to different pharmacodynamic models (Bonate, 2006; Macheras and Iliadis, 2006; Campbell, 1990; Yang et al., 2005).

Chapter 2

STOICHIOMETRY-BASED APPROACHES

I. GENERAL PRINCIPLES, CHARACTERISTICS AND APPLICATIONS OF STOICHIOMETRIC APPROACHES

Stoichiometric approaches elucidate systemic properties of cell metabolism by analysing the flux distributions space. This aim can be summarized around a key question: how the total flux within a cell will be distributed between the different chemical reactions or metabolic pathways under some considered constraints or experimental conditions (Figure 2.1)?

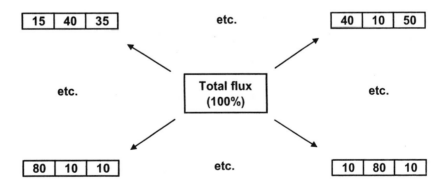

Figure 2.1. Illustration of different flux distributions among three components of metabolic system.

In flux analysis, the set of the factors governing a metabolic system are not known resulting in the absence of a unique target solution. Therefore, some constraints are considered to define (and refine) a feasible flux distribution space in which flux solutions can be determined. The definition and refinement of such a flux distribution space leads to (i) variation field location, (ii) shape determination and (iii) variation limits restriction. These three points are linked to three time-invariant constraints which can be mathematically expressed by means of equations or inequalities, describing steady-state flux distributions (i), flux irreversibility (ii) and system capacity (iii):

(i) The localisation of variation field of the flux distributions is initially defined by the steady-state (SS) or quasi-steady-state (qSS) assumption considering the metabolic system under a dynamical equilibrium between its input and output processes. SS represents a dynamical balance that the metabolic system reaches after a sufficient time leading to equilibrium between all the intracellular and extracellular fluxes (Figure 2.2). SS assumption avoids the difficulties in developing kinetic models due to the lack of intracellular measurements (Bailey, 1998; Palsson, 2000).

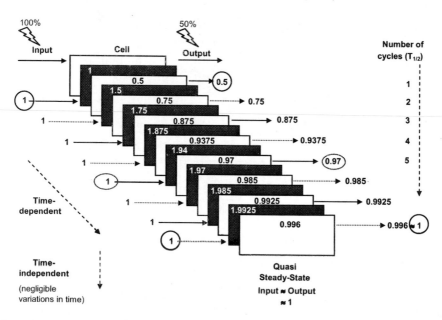

Figure 2.2. Succession of input-output processes leading to a steady-state (SS) in cell system after five input-output cycles. SS provides a reliable picture on a metabolic system. It is considered by stoichiometric analyses to overcome the difficulties due to lack of intracellular measurements and to kinetic models development.

Under SS constraint, the distribution of intracellular metabolic flux can be mathematically represented by the equation (1) :

$$S.v = 0 \qquad\qquad (2.1)$$

Where:

S: Known stoichiometric matrix of the metabolic system

v: Vector containing unknown (intracellular) fluxes to determine from a system of linear equations given by the matricial equation (2.1).

Geometrically, the set of all possible solutions of eq. (2.1) generates a space of flux distribution consisting of a hyperplane (Figure 2.3a).

(ii) The number of solutions can be reduced and the flux distribution space can be refined by imposing to the system a second invariant constraint consisting of flux irreversibility. Under such a constraint, all the flux are assumed to be unidirectional i.e. without reverse way. By convention, the natural flow direction is assigned to the positive direction. Mathematically, this constraint can be represented by the inequality:

$$v_j \geq 0 \qquad\qquad (2.2)$$

Where v_j is the flux or reaction j in metabolic system.

Geometrically, the combination of equation (2.1) with inequality (2.2) converts the hyperplane to a convex polyhedral cone (Figure 2.3b) (Price et al., 2004; Wagner and Urbanczik, 2005).

(iii) Convex polyhedral cone is well defined by its shape but has no upper borders. Upper limits can be defined by imposing to the system a third constraint consisting of capacity. System capacity bounds the convex polyhedral cone and transforms it into a polytope (Figure 2.3c). Mathematically, the capacity constraint can be expressed by the following inequality:

$$v_j \leq v_{max} \qquad\qquad (2.3)$$

Apart from these three invariant (non adjustable) constraints, adjustable constraints can be incorporated to further restrict the solution space of flux distributions helping to determine such fluxes or even to predict them (Covert et al., 2001; Schilling et al., 2002; Stelling et al., 2002).

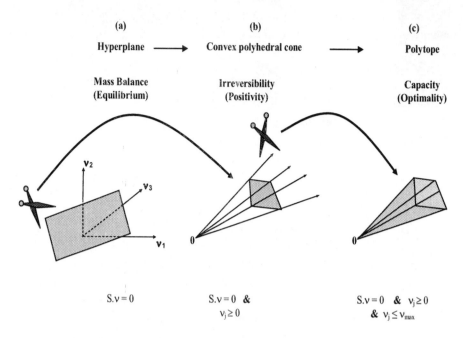

Figure 2.3. Three geometrical spaces of flux distributions defined by three time-invariant constraints consisting of steady state flux distributions (a), flux irreversibility (b) and system capacity (c).

Stoichiometric approaches represent powerful tools for metabolic modeling when time measurements are not available (Stephanopoulos et al., 1998). They make possible to exploit the knowledge about the organization of cell metabolism, without considering the intracellular kinetic processes (not directly accessible and still not well understood). Stoichiometric models are at the basis of different methods which have been used to (Llaneras and Picó, 2008; Morgan and Rhodes 2002; Stelling, 2004):

- Estimate the metabolic flux distribution under given static circumstances in the cell (metabolic flux analysis) (Williams et al., 2008; Ettenhuber et al., 2005; Kruger et al. 2003),
- Predict the metabolic flux distribution on the basis of some optimality hypotheses (flux balance analysis) (Schilling et al., 2001),
- Analyse systemic information on the topological organization of metabolic networks (pathway analysis) (Schilling et al., 1999, 2001).

II. METABOLIC FLUX ANALYSIS

II.1. General Concepts and Aim

Metabolic flux analysis (MFA) is a stoichiometric approach used to determine intracellular flux distributions between the different chemical reactions of metabolic networks. To this aim, three basic knowledge points are needed:

- Measured extracellular fluxes.
- Stoichiometric coefficients of all the chemical reactions of the metabolic network.
- Steady state constraint assuming null intracellular flux variations due to a balance between input and output of the metabolic system.

By opposition to intracellular fluxes, extracellular fluxes can be easily measured leading to gain information on the system. The intracellular fluxes represent unknown parameters and will be determined by a set of linear equations issued from the SS general equation S.v=0 (Eq. 2.1).

Initially the system is underdetermined because the number of its unknown fluxes (parameters to determine) is generally higher than the number of its metabolites (equations to solve). To offset the undeterminacy of the system defined by Eq. 2.1, a sufficient number of extracellular fluxes (of initial substrates and final products) will be experimentally measured then used in Eq. 2.1 to mathematically determine the unknown intracellular fluxes (Llaneras and Picó, 2008). If need, additional constraints can be incorporated to reduce the system dimensionality. In general, the system defined by Eq. 2.1. is determined when there are sufficient linearly independent constraints to uniquely calculate all unmeasured fluxes v_j of the intracellular reactions j.

II.2. Principles and Methodology

The methodology of MFA can be summarized into three steps (Figure 2.4):

1) Initially, the metabolic map of all the metabolites interconnected by all the chemical reactions needs to be established.

2) Then, such metabolic map will be represented by a stoichiometric
    matrix combined with a flux vector separating intracellular and
    extracellular spaces:

Stoichiometric matrix gives stoichiometric coefficients representing the
numbers of molecules of metabolites consumed and produced by the different
chemical reactions. In a stoichiometric matrix, the rows are metabolites, the
columns are chemical reactions and the inside values are stoichiometric
coefficients (Figure 1.9). Such coefficients are invariant (time-independent)
properties of the metabolic system. Positive and negative coefficients represent
production and consumption processes, respectively.

Apart from the stoichiometric coefficients which define the invariant
chemical behavior of the system, the fluxes of the different reactions are
needed to consider the metabolic variability of such a system: although the
chemical reactions are stoichiometrically invariant, they can be more or less
invested according to different regulation processes (enzyme activities, gene
expressions, etc.). Therefore, the behavior of metabolic system is *a priori*
defined by a combination between the stoichiometric matrix S and a flux
vector v.

Finally, in this second step, the cellular space is divided into extracellular
and intracellular. Being experimentally accessible, the extracellular fluxes are
measured then used to mathematical determination of the intracellular fluxes
(non accessible experimentally).

3) In a third step, the metabolic system is considered under SS
    constraint, and its unknown intracellular fluxes will be determined by
    solving the general equation (2.1) detailed in figure 2.5.

The determination of intracellular fluxes from Eq. (2.1) will help to
understand how the fluxes were distributed in the metabolic map linking initial
substrates to final products.

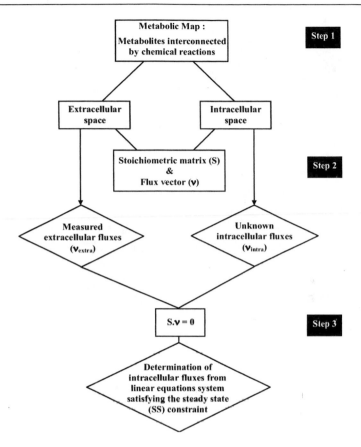

Figure 2.4. Different methodological steps in metabolic flux analysis (MFA)

$$known \dashrightarrow \begin{Bmatrix} S_{intra} \\ S_{extra} \end{Bmatrix} \cdot v = \begin{pmatrix} 0 \\ v' \end{pmatrix} \dashleftarrow \begin{array}{l} \text{Steady state constraint} \\ \text{Measured experimentally} \end{array}$$

to predict

$$\Leftrightarrow$$

$$v = \left[\begin{pmatrix} S_{int\,ra} \\ S_{extra} \end{pmatrix}' \begin{pmatrix} S_{int\,ra} \\ S_{extra} \end{pmatrix} \right]^{-1} \begin{pmatrix} S_{int\,ra} \\ S_{extra} \end{pmatrix}' \begin{pmatrix} 0 \\ v' \end{pmatrix}$$

Figure 2.5. Illustrated computation of the intracellular flux vector v from the development of equation (2.1). S_{intra} and S_{extra}: matrices of intracellular and extracellular stoichiometric coefficients, respectively; v': vector of measured extracellular fluxes.

II.3. Application Example

To illustrate the three steps of MFA and its result interpretation, let's give a simple example of a metabolic network containing 6 metabolites interconnected by 6 chemical reactions (Figure 2.6):

1) From the knowledge of the metabolic map, the six metabolites can be separated into three intracellular (intermediate metabolites A, B, C) and three extracellular including two substrates (S1, S2) and one final product P1 (Figure 2.6a).

2) The reactions interconnecting all the metabolites are stored into a stoichiometric matrix S in which intracellular and extracellular metabolites are well distinct (Figure 2.6b). The invariant stoichiometric coefficients interact with different variable fluxes v_j leading to different possible flux distributions in the metabolic system. The six fluxes v_1-v_6 are stored into a flux vector v. The extracellular fluxes (v_1, v_3, v_4) are measured then used to mathematically determine the three unknown fluxes v_2, v_5, v_6.

3) The interactions between stoichiometric coefficients and the metabolic fluxes can be mathematically translated by the product of the stoichiometric matrix S with the flux vector v: S.v . Under the steady state (SS) constraint, this product is puted to zero concerning the intracellular space, i.e. $S_{intra}.v = 0$ (Figure 2.6c). For the measured (known) extracellular fluxes, their values will be affected by positive or negative signs in the product $S_{extra}.v$: negative fluxes are associated to the substrates S1 and S2 (disappearance) (-v_1, -v_4); positive fluxes are associated to the product P1 (appearance) (+v_3).

The resulting system of 3 equations with 3 unknowns shows null determinant meaning infinity of possible solutions satisfying the SS situation (Figure 2.6d). Particular solutions can be determined by attributing a given value to an intracellular flux to determine how the others will be distributed (Figure 2.6e):

   i)   Thus for v_5=1, v_2 and v_6 will be equal to 5 and 1, respectively. Such intracellular flux distribution shows equilibrated fluxes between the reaction C→A and C→B, and a major flux oriented from A to B.

   ii)   In the case where the flux v_2 is minor (=1), the most flux distribution is expected to concern the reaction C→B more favorable to product P1 (v_6=6), whereas the flux of reaction C→A shows a negative value (v_5=-3): this can indicate that metabolite A must be transformed to C to satisfy the flux demand of reaction C→B; however, such interpretation is valid only under possible flux reversibility.

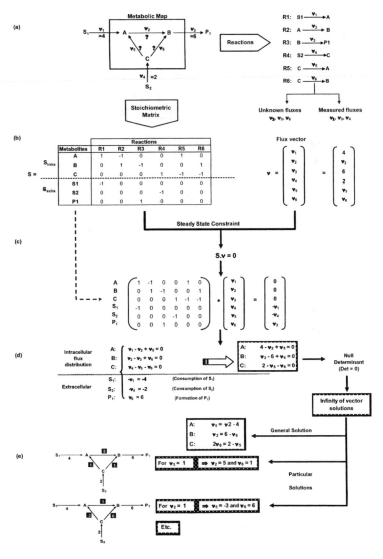

Figure 2.6. Application example illustrating the metabolic flux analysis.

II.4. Application Fields of MFA

MFA has different interests in biological sciences and medical fields. It was applied to:

- Characterize canonical states of cells such as exponential growth or steady states in the continuous culture modes (Fisher et al., 2004; Wiechert et al., 2001; Bonarius et al., 1996; Follstad et al., 1999; Nyberg et al., 1999; Gambhir et al., 2003; Schwender et al., 2004; Ratcliffe et al., 2006; Lange, 2006, Shimizu, 2002).
- Study transient processes in microorganisms (Herwig and von Stockar, 2002).
- On-line monitoring of intracellular fluxes in mammalian cells (Takiguchi et al., 1997).
- Optimize extracellular bioartificial liver device (Sharma et al., 2005).

III. METABOLIC PATHWAY ANALYSIS

III.1. General Concepts and Aim

Metabolic pathway analysis (MPA) aims at the elucidation of systemic properties emerging from the entire metabolic network. Such properties are extracted by considering the network as a set of metabolic pathways (MPs). MPs are high functional units in metabolic systems linking initial substrates to final products through serials of chemical reactions working in same directions (Klamt and Stelling, 2003; Papin et al., 2003, 2004; Schuster and Hilgetag, 1994; Trinh et al., 2009).

Identification of MPs represents a major aim to understand functional organizations and evolutive aspects of metabolic networks. MPs are identified on the basis of some functional and mathematical independence criteria leading to two types of pathways called elementary modes (i) and extreme pathways (ii):

i) Functional independence means non-reductible or non-decomposable pathways (Figure 2.7), i.e. a MP that can't be reduced to a simpler route (Schuster and Hilgetag, 1994; Schilling et al., 1999; Schuster et al., 1999). The functional non-decomposability is can be checked when the entire pathway becomes inactive if any of its flux is put to zero (Schuster and Hilgetag, 1994; Schuster et al., 2002a, 2002b; Pfeiffer et al., 1999). Subsequently, MPs contain minimum numbers of chemical reactions linking initial substrates to corresponding final products. Such functionally irreductible pathways are called elementary modes (EMs). They are stoichiometrically and thermodynamically feasible routes to the conversion of substrates into products. They can also be associated to independent expressions of the genetic system by the fact that each EM contains a different set of functional genes that can support cellular function at steady state (Trinh et al., 2009).

ii)   Beyond the functional independence represented by EMs, the number of MPs in a metabolic system can be further reduced by considering mathematical or linear independence: although EMs are functionally independent, some of them can be mathematically obtained from linear combinations of others (Figure 2.7). By subtracting the non-linearly independent EMs from the total number of EMs, one obtains the extreme pathways (EPs). In other words, none EP can be obtained by a non-negative combination of at least two other EPs (Klamt and Stelling, 2003; Schilling et al., 2000; Papin et al., 2003, 2004).

After identification of EMs and EPs, their flux distributions can be analysed by elementary mode analysis (EMA) and extreme pathway analysis (EPA), respectively. This helps to interpret the overall capabilities of cell metabolism from a finite basic set of flux distributions (flux vectors) representing the systemic properties of the system.

III.2. Principles and Methodology

Identification of EMs in a metabolic network is carried out taking into account three time-invariant (non-adjustable) constraints:

- Steady state flux distribution (mass balance): $S.v=0$
- Flux irreversibility (thermodynamic feasibility): $v \geq 0$
- Non decomposability of pathways (functional or genetic independence)

Identification of EPs among all the EMs requires a fourth non-adjustable constraint consisting of systematic independence (linear independence) of the pathways.

EMs and EPs represent time-invariant properties of metabolic systems as they are identified on the basis of non-adjustable constraints.

Geometrically, the two first constraints (SS and irreversibility) restrict the set of possible SS flux distributions to a convex polyhedral cone (Figure 2.3) (Rockafellar, 1970). The third constraint (functional independence) defines EMs within the convex space as vectors e_k originated from chained flux routes covering all the expressions of metabolic system. Such vectors might lie on the surface or the interior of the convex space (Figure 2.7).

From the q identified EMs (e_k), any SS flux distribution v in the metabolic system can be obtained by a linear combination with non-negative coefficients λ_k of e_k:

$$v = \sum_{k=1}^{q} \lambda_k e_k = \lambda_1 e_1 + \ldots + \lambda_q e_q$$

$$(2.4)$$

Where:

$\lambda_k \geq 0$ ($k=1$ to q) could be defined as the "activity" of the EM (e_k).The number q defines the dimension of the convex polyhedral cone.

By incorporating the fourth constraint (linear independence) to the three previous ones, the number of identified EMs will be reduced to EPs representing the minimal number w ($w \leq q$) of flux vectors that can be linearly combined with non-negative coefficients to generate all the other fluxes in the convex space. EPs correspond to a subset of EMs representing the unique and minimal set needed to describe all allowable SS flux distributions through the metabolic network (Figure 2.7) (Schilling et al., 2000). For instance, figure 2.7 shows that EM4 is not EP because it can be obtained by combining EM1 and EM2. However EM1-EM3 represent the three EPs of the system.

Geometrically, EPs are the edges of convex polyhedral cone (Figure 2.7).

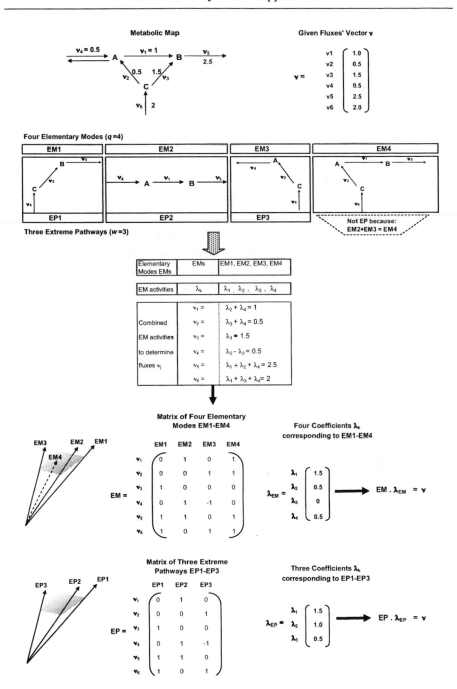

Figure 2.7. Illustrative example of elementary mode and extreme pathway analyses.

III.3. Application Fields of MPA

MPA allows a systematic and objective evaluation of metabolism capabilities in terms of cellular robustness, fragility and regulation. It doesn't require any knowledge on external (measured) flux or objective function for cellular metabolism.

In plant sciences, EMA has been applied by Poolman et al. (2003) to show that Calvin cycle and oxidative pentose phosphate pathway are, in the context of chloroplast, complementary and overlapping components of the same system. The structural properties of the plant mitochondrial TCA cycle have also been described using EMA (Steuer et al., 2007).

In biomedical sciences, EMA was applied to analyse the metabolism of cultured hepatocytes in extracorporeal bioartificial liver devices (Zhong, 2002), and to investigate the metabolic responses of the rat liver to burn-injury-induced whole body inflammation (Nolan et al., 2006). EPA was applied to better understand the human red blood cell metabolism (Wiback and Palsson, 2002).

In microbiology, EMA and EPA were applied in the context of metabolic productions of *Escherichia coli* (Schmidt et al., 1999; Van-Dien et al., 2006), *Heamophilus influenzae* (Schilling and Palsson, 2000; Papin et al., 2002) and *H. pylori* (Price et al., 2002). EPs were used to classify chemical reactions into groups that are always, sometimes or never utilized for the production of a target product (Papin et al., 2002): Comparisons of distributions of EP lengths between *Heliobacter pylori* and *Haemophilus influenzae* revealed systemic differences between the two microorganisms, despite overall similar metabolic networks. Pathway analysis was also applied to identify the function of orphane genes in the yeast *Saccharomyces cerevisiae* (Förster et al., 2002).

IV. FLUX BALANCE ANALYSIS

IV.1. General Concepts and Aim

Flux balance analysis (FBA) aims at finding intracellular flux distributions or extracellular conditions which optimize objective biological functions (Lee et al., 2006). Such optimization includes maximization of biomass, ATP or metabolite production, minimization of ATP consumption, etc. Apart from optimal intracellular flux distributions, FBA helps to find combinations of extracellular substrates that optimize well defined biological functions.

IV.2. Principles and Methodology

FBA is applied under the fundamental assumption that cell is able to achieve optimal behaviors in its biological activities with respect to certain objectives.

Optimization in FBA is carried out by considering three invariant constraints combined with some variant (adjustable) input constraint(s) (Figure 2.8). Invariant constraints assume:

- Steady state fluxes (mass balance constraint): $S.v=0$
- Flux irreversibility: $v \geq 0$
- Flux capacity : $v \leq v_{max}$

These three constraints define the space of optimal flux distribution as a bounded convex space: the incorporation of the third constraint (capacity) converts the convex polyhedral cone to a bounded convex polytope (Figure 2.3).

The unknown optimal flux vector v satisfying the three invariant constraints is combined with a vector c of controllable input constraints consisting of coefficients or weights of the fluxes in v (Beard et al., 2002). This leads to mathematical formulation of a linear objective function Z to optimize:

$$Z = c.v = \sum_{j=1}^{p} c_j . v_j \tag{2.5}$$

From this linear combination where the elements of c can be adjusted, different objective biological functions Z can be considered: the key of FBA is to figure out what objective functions likely represent the cellular metabolism under a given growth condition (Schuetz et al., 2007). Therefore, the function Z will be maximized or minimized leading to determine the flux distribution (flux vector v) that satisfies the optimization problem. Optimal solution of Z can be solved with linear programming (Strang, 1986). However, it should be mentioned that FBA identifies only one optimal solution while alternative optimal solutions or suboptimal ones can exist.

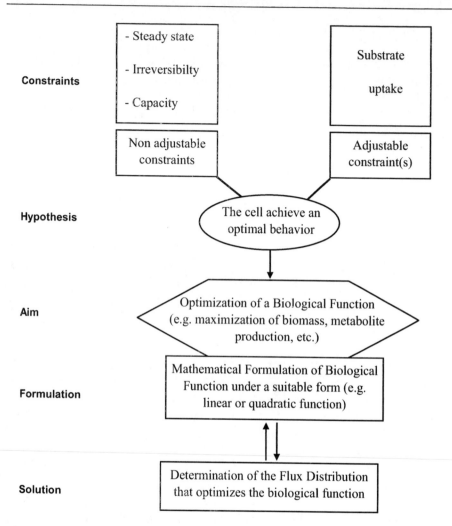

Figure 2.8. General principles of flux balance analysis (FBA).

FBA can be applied to determine a metabolic flux vector **v** of a cellular physiological state when knowledge of extracellular fluxes is limited and intracellular stoichiometric matrix cannot be inverted to provide unique solution. For that FBA requires specification of objective functions representing correctly the cellular metabolism. Anyhow, the more fluxes can be measured, the more accurately the flux vector can be computationally determined.

IV.3. Application Fields of FBA

Many applications of FBA have been investigated including (Palsson, 2006; Edwards et al., 2002; Price et al., 2003; Shimizu, 2002): identification and prioritization of candidate drug targets, simulation of gradual inhibition, analysis of enzyme deficiencies, prediction of behavior under knockout conditions, etc. The last case can be illustrated by the prediction of metabolic flux vectors of knockout genes by imposing the constraint that mutants operate by optimizing their metabolic adjustments with respect to the wild type (Serge et al., 2002).

Chapter 3

CORRELATION-BASED APPROACHES

I. GENERAL AIMS

Relationships between variables can be undertaken by correlation analysis which takes into account the dispersions, global inclinations and shapes of data. Correlation analysis leads to quantify the reciprocal effect of two variables each on the other. For that, different statistical parameters are calculated, viz. correlation coefficients, confidence ranges, slopes, etc. Correlation coefficient quantifies the monotony degree of relationship between variables, but it provides no information on the kind of their relationship. Moreover, correlation coefficient gives some qualitative information on the direction or inclination of relationship through its sign: positive or negative signs indicate increasing or decreasing trends, respectively. The inclination of the cloud of points representing the dataset is quantified by the slope of the statistical model used to describe the data variability. The model is defined by an equation which is used to fit the shape of the cloud of points. The most commonly used model is the linear model represented by the equation $y=ax+b$. Several other models can be used according to the shape of cloud of points (y vs x), viz. logarithmic ($y=Ln(x)$), square root ($y=\sqrt{x}$), inverse ($y=1/x$), exponential ($y=e^x$). These models are applied on curvilinear clouds of points to bring data linearization leading to benefit from computation and simplicity advantages of the linear model. Beyond these transformations applicable to specific data shapes, the general Box-Cox transformation is a family of power transformations aiming at the determination of exponent which give close-normality and homoscedasticity data (Box and Cox, 1964; Box et al., 1978).

II. METHODOLOGICAL STEPS IN CORRELATION ANALYSIS

II.1. Graphical Identification of Correlation Models

The first step in correlation analysis consists in visualizing the bivariate data by means of naïve scatter plots. One obtains clouds of points from which the relationships between variables (e.g. metabolites) can be described by dispersions, inclinations and shapes (Figure 3.1).

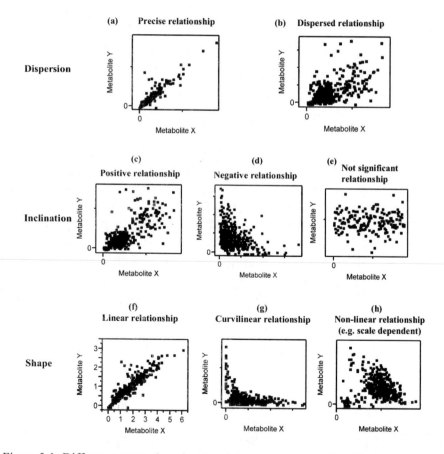

Figure 3.1. Different scatter plots showing different characteristics (dispersion, inclination, shape) from which statistical tools can be appropriately used to quantify and to fit relationships between variables (e.g. metabolites).

For thin or few dispersed and well stretched clouds of points (Figure 3.1a, f), relationships between variables can be quantified by means of Pearson correlation coefficient. In the case of more dispersed data (Figure 3.1b-d, h), Spearman correlation coefficient can be used as robust statistic to detect trends between variables (metabolites). Positive (Figure 3.1a-c, f) and negative (Figure 3.1d, g) relationships will be indicated by positive and negative correlation coefficients, respectively.

Pearson correlation is sensitive to the non-linearity of data (Figure 3.1d, g, h). In the case of curvilinear relationships, the use of Pearson coefficient can find application after data linearization using appropriate transformations. Appropriate transformations provide symmetrical distributions (close to normal) of the data by reducing their dispersion, asymmetry and bias effects of isolated (extreme) points (Zar, 1999). Such transformations can be applied either on only one or on both variables of the pair (X, Y).

Moreover, such transformations are applied to stabilize the variances between several groups of the dataset, i.e. in the case of heteroscedastic data (non comparable variances between groups). Therefore, the resulting homoscedasticity will make possible the application of linear model.

II.2. Preliminary Data Transformations to Linear Model Application

From a graphical visualization, a curvilinear cloud of points (Y vs X) can be transformed into linear form by using an appropriate formula (Zar, 1999, Legendre and Legendre, 2000). Such a formula depends on the shape, intensity of curvature and number of inflexion point(s) of the cloud of points Y vs X (Figure 3.2).

Logarithmic transformations are appropriate to linearize curvature showing slow (i) or accelerated (ii) variations of Y vs X after an inflection (Figure 3.3). In the first case (i) (Figure 3.3a), linearization is obtained from Y vs $Ln(X)$; in the second case (ii) (Figure 3.3b), linearization is obtained from $Ln(Y)$ vs X. More precisely, the fonction $Y = a\,e^{bX}$ is linearized by taking the log of Y to give a straight-line equation with intercept $\ln(a)$ and slope b, i.e. $\ln(Y) = \ln(a) + bX$. In the case where Y and X are linked by a power function $Y=a(X)^c$, such a non-linear relationship can be linearized by taking the logarithms of both X and Y, giving linear equation $\ln(Y) = \ln(a) + c\,\ln(X)$ (Figure 3.3c). In general, from a curvilinear cloud of points, the appropriate model can be identified from the transformation by which the curve becomes aligned (Figure 3.3).

Taking into account the distribution of each variable, logarithmic transformation can be applied to a right asymmetric distribution, i.e. having a mode located at the left (a majority of low values). Therefore, logarithmic transformation results in more symmetrical distribution, i.e. a distribution closer to normality conditions making a possible application of the linear model (Figure 3.4).

Square root transformation can be applied to linearize parabolic cloud of points. Moreover, the square root can be preferred to the logarithm transformation (more generally used) in the case of small dataset (few number of observations). Graphically, models requiring square root transformation have more soft curvature than those requiring logarithmic transformation (Figure 3.2a).

Clouds of points can be also linearized by means of polynomial transformations. This is generally applied in the case where different inflexion points are observed: a cloud with k inflexion points can be fitted by means of a polynome with a degree $(k+1)$ (Figure 3.2d).

II.3. Correlation Coefficient Computation

The correlation concept is used to analyze the dependency between two variables (metabolites). The dependency degree between variables is quantified by a correlation coefficient having two aspects: its absolute value and its sign. Absolute value of correlation coefficient varies between 0 and 1; a higher value indicates a stronger dependency degree between the variables. All the same, small correlation values can be statistically significant when a great number of points confirm it. This can be observed in large datasets containing many repeated experimental measurements. On the other hand, some high correlations can be not significant because they are calculated on few data.

The sign of correlation indicates if the two variables vary simultaneously in the same sense or if they are opposite: positive and negative correlation coefficients indicate increasing (affinity) and decreasing (opposition) relationships between the variables, respectively.

Different correlation coefficients can be calculated according to the dataset structure:

- Pearson correlation coefficient is calculated under the assumptions of data normality and linearity (Zar, 1999). It is a parametric correlation coefficient, and thus, it is calculated directly from the measured values (e.g. concentrations). Under normality and linearity conditions, Pearson correlation has the advantage to conserve a maximum of information from the dataset, making it to be a more powerful procedure compared to Spearman's.
- Spearman correlation coefficient requires neither linearity nor normality. It is a non-parametric coefficient calculated on the ranks of sorted values. It can be applied to detect trends between variables, and it is especially interesting in the case of sparse datasets. The fact that Spearman correlation doesn't depend on linearity but only monotonicity, makes it to be more robust than Pearson correlation toward the outliers (Spearman, 1904; Zar, 1999).

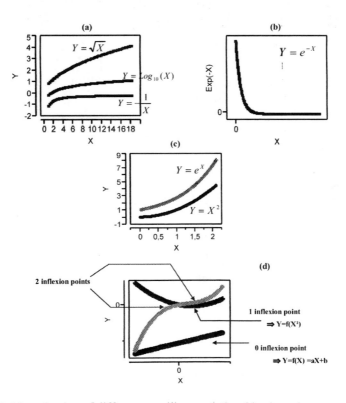

Figure 3.2. Linearization of different curvilinear relationships by using appropriate data transformations.

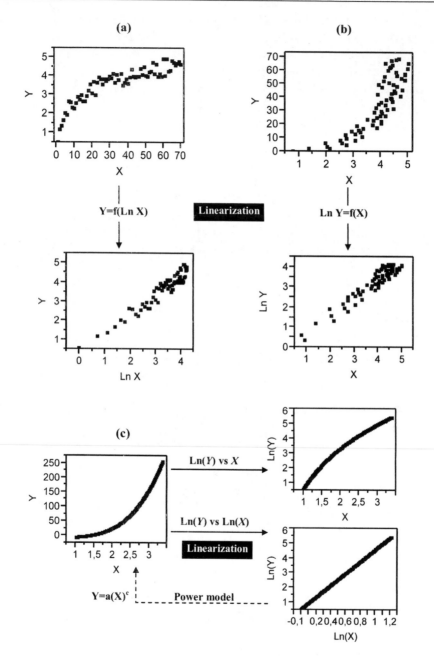

Figure 3.3. Applications of logarithmic transformations to data linearization.

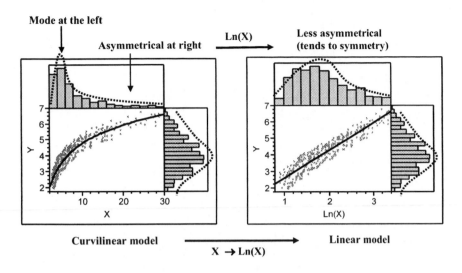

Figure 3.4. Logarithmic transformation attenuating right asymmetric distribution to be close to normality conditions (necessary to linear model application).

II.3.1. Pearson Correlation Computation

Pearson correlation coefficient (r) between two variables x and y is calculated by using the following formula tacking into account their variances and covariance:

$$r = \frac{C_{xy}}{S_x \cdot S_y} = \frac{\dfrac{\sum_{i=1}^{n}(x_i - \overline{x})(y_i - \overline{y})}{n-1}}{\sqrt{\dfrac{\sum_{i=1}^{n}(x_i - \overline{x})^2}{n-1}} \cdot \sqrt{\dfrac{\sum_{i=1}^{n}(y_i - \overline{y})^2}{n-1}}} = \frac{\sum_{i=1}^{n}(x_i - \overline{x})(y_i - \overline{y})}{\sqrt{\sum_{i=1}^{n}(x_i - \overline{x})^2} \cdot \sqrt{\sum_{i=1}^{n}(y_i - \overline{y})^2}} \qquad (3.1)$$

where:

C_{xy} is the covariance of the variables x and y

S_x and S_y: are the standard deviations of x and y

x_i and y_i are measured values (concentration values) of the variables x and y, respectively, in individual i

$\overline{x}$ and $\overline{y}$ are the means of the variables x and y, respectively.

n is the number of paired values (x_i, y_i), i.e. the total number of individuals (rows) i in the dataset.

Let's give a numerical example to illustrate the calculation of Pearson correlation (Figure 3.5). Suppose we have a metabolic dataset (10 rows × 4 columns) describing 10 profiles by the concentrations of 4 metabolites:

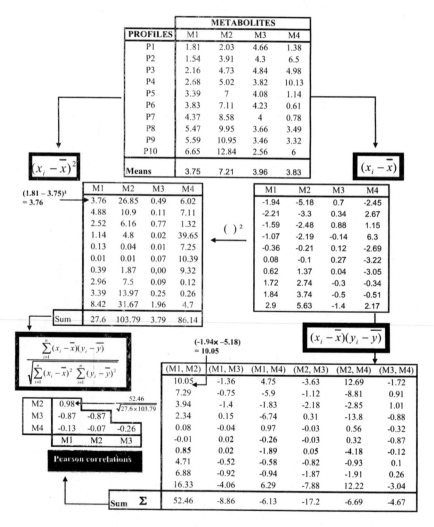

Figure 3.5. Computation of Pearson correlations between four variables (e.g. metabolites) M1, M2, M3, M4 from a dataset of 10 individuals (e.g. 10 concentration profiles).

One obtains six correlation values ($0 \leq r \leq 1$) varying by their absolute values and their signs. The highest correlation value concerns the pair of metabolites (M_1, M_2) (+0.98), whereas the lowest concerns (M_2, M_4) (-0.07). Metabolite M_4 appears to be the less correlated to all the others. From the signs of correlations, metabolite M_3 appears to be strongly negatively correlated to M_1 and M_2 ($r_{1,3}$=-0.87 and $r_{2,3}$=-0.87). In addition to their quantification by Pearson coefficients, the correlations can be qualitatively analyzed by graphical visualization of the clouds of points (Figure 3.6).

The scatter plot matrix shows that the strong positive correlation between M_1 and M_2 was due to a thin (few dispersed) monotonous cloud of points. The absolute values of correlations decrease with the dispersions of the clouds of points; such dispersions can be represented by confidence ellipse thicknesses. This is well illustrated by the lowest correlations between M_4 and the other metabolites where the dispersed variation spaces show spherical shapes instead of elliptic. Such spherical shapes can be interpreted by absences of linearity between the variables.

After correlation computations, conclusions will be finally established by testing the significance of each correlation. Two variables (metabolites) will be concluded to be linked if their correlation coefficient is statistically significant. Pearson correlations are tested by using the Student t statistics calculated by reference to the value zero (r=0). The null value represents absence of correlation, and therefore the test will respond to the question: does the tested correlation r is significantly different from 0 or no?. The Student test consists in calculating a standardized value t of r:

$$t = \frac{|r - 0|}{s_r} \qquad (3.2)$$

The standard deviation s_r of the correlation coefficient r is calculated by the following formula:

$$s_r = \sqrt{\frac{1 - r^2}{n - 2}} \qquad (3.3)$$

where n is the number of measurements (rows, individuals, profiles). Therefore the formula of t can be written:

$$t = \left| \frac{r\sqrt{n-2}}{\sqrt{1-r^2}} \right|$$ (3.4)

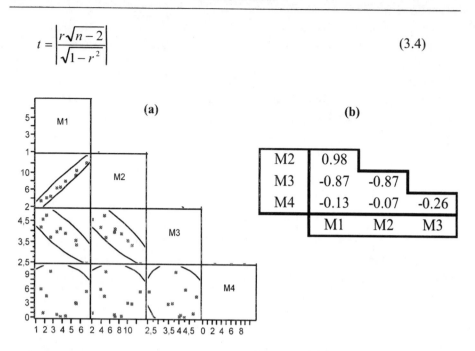

Figure 3.6. (a) Scatter plot matrix showing the variations between different variables (metabolite concentrations); (b) Correlation matrix corresponding to the scatter plot matrix presented in (a).

The calculated t value will be compared to a cut-off value given by the Student table for a low risk α (e.g. 0.05 = 5%) and a degree of freedom df=n-2 (Figure 3.7). A correlation coefficient r will be concluded to be significant if its calculated statistics t_{cal} is higher than the tabulated cut off value $t_{tab}(\alpha, n\text{-}2)$. In such a case, one concludes that r is statistically significant (significantly different from 0) with a fail risk $\leq \alpha$. If $t_{cal} < t_{tab}(\alpha, n\text{-}2)$, one concludes that r is not significantly different from 0 at the considered level α.

The results show that the correlation correlations are significantly different from 0 with α risk $\leq 5\%$ for the pairs (M_1, M_2), (M_1, M_3) and (M_2, M_3). However, the correlations between M_4 and M_1, M_2, M_3 were not significantly different from 0 at the α level = 5%.

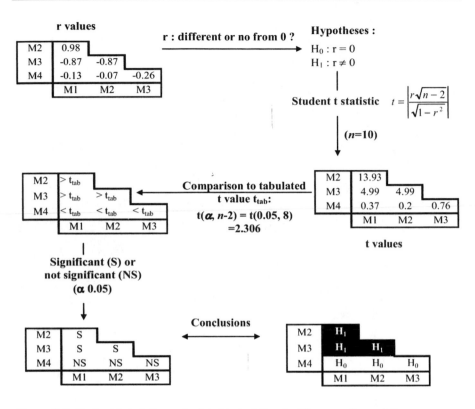

Figure 3.7. Student t statistics calculated to test the significance of correlation coefficients.

II.3.2. Matrix Correlation Computation

Generally, experimental datasets (e.g. metabolomic datasets) contain more variables than the simple illustrative example of figure 3.5. Therefore, it becomes useful to handle information and to carry out calculation directly by means of matricial tools leading to avoid time-consuming repeated calculus. Pearson correlation matrix of a dataset (n rows $\times$ p columns) can be calculated by a single product between the standardized data matrix S and its transposed S' ($S'S$), divided by the degree of freedom (n-1) (Figure 3.8) (Legendre and Legendre, 2000). A numerical example is given in Figure 3.9.

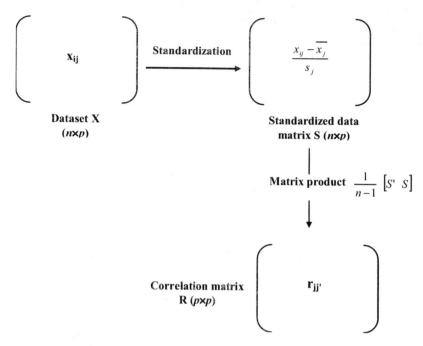

Figure 3.8. Principle of correlation matrix computation.

II.3.3. Spearman Correlation Calculation

Spearman coefficient is a non parametric coefficient which requires less conditions than the parametric Pearson coefficient. It can be calculated without to have to check or to assume normality, homoscedasticity and linearity of/between variables. However, the number n of individuals must be higher to 10 to be able to test the significance of Spearman correlation. In other words, the use of Spearman correlation is advised for datasets with great number of measures. This is all the more since such datasets have generally high dispersions from which significant trends can be reliably identified by Spearman correlation. If either Spearman or Pearson correlation analysis is applicable (checked application conditions), the former is $9/\pi^2 = 0.91$ as powerful as the later (Daniel, 1978; Hotelling and Pabst, 1936). The significance of calculated Spearman rank correlations are accessed by consulting statistical tables giving cut-off values in relation to the number of measurements n and α level.

Spearman correlation is calculated on the ranks of values and not on the values themselves. For that, its calculation requires *a priori* the ranking of the values x_i, y_i of variables x, y. This operation is different from sorting because the different values are maintained at their respective positions, but are just replaced by numbers which gives their position ranks. The values corresponding to minimum and maximum of each variable will have the ranks 1 and n, respectively. All the other values will have intermediate ranks. Finally, the association degree between the ranks of the two variables is then quantified by using the Spearman correlation coefficient ρ (Zar, 1999):

$$\rho = 1 - \frac{6\sum_{i=1}^{n} d_i^2}{n^3 - n} \qquad (3.5)$$

Where :

   d_i is the difference between the ranks of x_i and y_i values.
   n is the number of paired values.

   The computation of Spearman correlations (ρ) is illustrated by a numerical example consisting of a dataset of 12 rows ($n>10$) and 4 columns (Figure 3.10). We suppose we have a concentration dataset of 4 metabolites analysed in 12 individuals to obtain 12 concentration profiles (in arbitrary unit).

   The calculated ρ values show positive correlations between metabolites M_1, M_2 and M_3, and negative correlations between these three metabolites and M_4. A statistical table gives for $\alpha=0.05$ and $n=12$, a tabulated value $\rho_{tab}=0.587$, leading to conclude that there are four significant correlations with α risk $\leq 5\%$ (M_1-M_2; M_1-M_3; M_2-M_3; M_3-M_4), against two not significant at α level $= 5\%$ (M_1-M_4; M_2-M_4) (from ρ absolute values). From the scatter plot matrix (Figure 3.11a), the significant correlations correspond to thin and sharply inclined clouds of points, whereas the not significant ones correspond to weakly inclined clouds of points (nearly horizontal; Figure 3.1e). Note that the significant negative correlation between M_3 and M_4 corresponds also to a weakly inclined cloud, but which is less dispersed (thin confidence ellipse) than the pairs (M_1, M_4) and (M_2, M_4). This shows that a correlation coefficient takes into account both the covariance (inclination) and the variance (dispersion) of the variables.

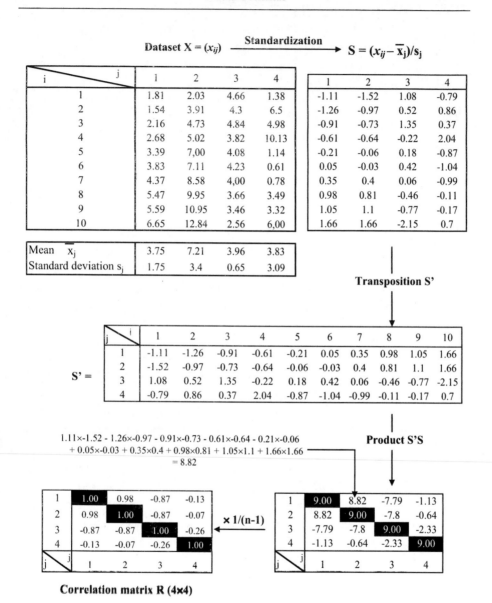

Figure 3.9. Numerical example illustrating the computation of Pearson correlation matrix from a standardized dataset.

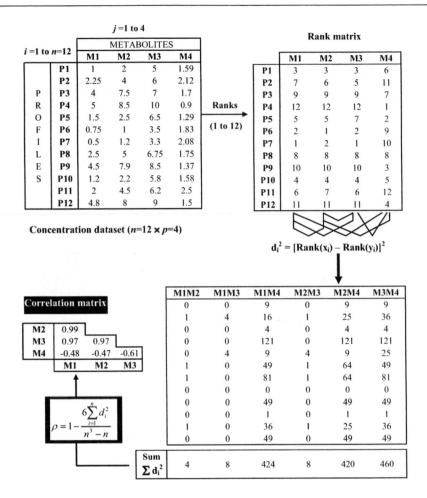

Figure 3.10. Numerical example illustrating the computation of Spearman correlations (ρ) between paired variables.

As the correlations were calculated on concentrations, they have to be interpreted in terms of biosynthesis or by reference to control processes of substrates' availability, because the concentration is all the more high since the biosynthesis or absorption process is important. On this basis, significantly positive correlations between M_1, M_2 and M_3 can be indicative of common factors favoring the biosyntheses (common metabolic pathways, common resources, sensitivity toward same stimulus factors, same cell transport paths, etc.). Concerning the pair (M_3, M_4), its significantly negative correlation can be originated from different situations, such as metabolites which:

i)   have opposite characteristics (e.g. biosynthesis and
        elimination which are rapid for one metabolite and slow for
        the other),

ii) belong to two alternative or lagged metabolic pathways,

iii) are stimulated by different (not shared) factors, etc. .

Finally, the not significant correlations of M_4 toward M_1 and M_2 indicate
that there are not sufficient oriented factors/characteristics to group or to
opposite these metabolites.

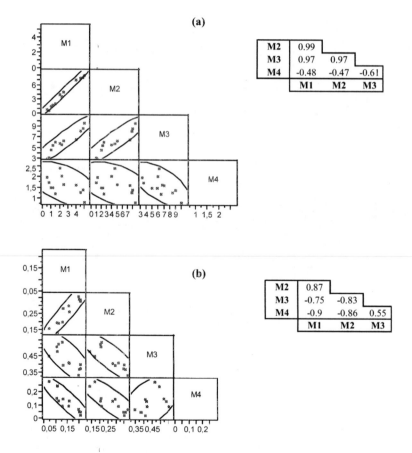

Figure 3.11. Scatter plots and correlation matrices providing a visualization and
quantification of relationships between concentrations (a) and relative levels (b) of
different variables M_1, M_2, M_3, M_4.

Apart from the concentration variables which are directly interpretable in terms of synthesis or availability, metabolomics focuses on the analysis of the relative levels of such concentrations which are interpretable in terms of metabolic regulation ratios. Regulation ratios of different metabolites provide information on the internal organization of their metabolic systems, whereas concentrations are particularly appropriate to analyse the metabolic machine in relation to external conditions.

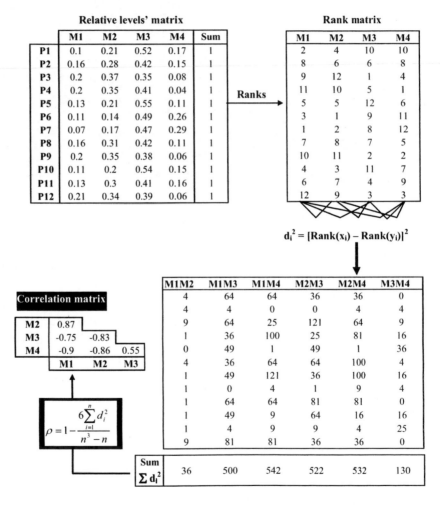

Figure 3.12. Numerical example illustrating the computation of Spearman correlations (ρ) between regulation ratio variables.

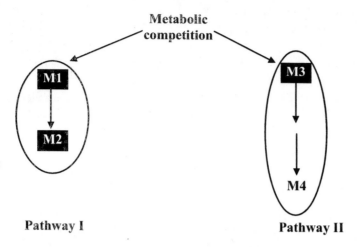

Figure 3.13. Hypothetic scheme on the global organization of metabolic system interpreted from Spearman correlations between relative levels of metabolites (M_1, M_2, M_3, M_4). Black squares (M_1-M_3) indicate metabolites sharing some factors favoring their biosynthesis, and interpreted from correlations between their concentrations (rather than relative levels). Double arrow between M_3 and M_4 is indicative of a lesser neighboring between them, interpreted from a lower absolute value of correlation between their relative levels.

Spearman correlations can be calculated on relative level data to evaluate links between regulation ratios of different metabolites. Such a computation is illustrated from the relative levels of concentration data previously presented in figure 3.10.

Five among the six correlation values are significant with $\alpha \leq 5\%$, because they are higher than the cut off tabulated value $\rho_{tab}=0.587$ ($\alpha=0.05$ and $n=12$) (Figure 3.12) (Figure 3.11b). Although at α level of 5%, the positive correlation 0.55 is not significant, it is enough high to be considered as significant with α risk $\leq 10\%$ ($\rho_{tab}(\alpha=10\%, n=12)=0.503$) (Zar, 1999).

From positive and negative correlations, the four compounds are organized into two subsets each one containing positively correlated metabolites: M_1, M_2 on the hand, and M_3, M_4 on the other hand. The compounds of each subset are negatively correlated to those of the other subset (Figure 3.11b). The negative correlations can be indicative of the presence of two competitive metabolic pathways (M_1, M_2) against (M_3, M_4). In other words, the metabolic regulations of M_1, M_2 occur at the expense of M_3, M_4, and vice versa. From the positive correlations, the value of the pair (M_1, M_2) which is higher (and more significant) than that of (M_3, M_4) can be indicative of more shared factors (metabolic processes, chemical structure similarities, etc) between M_1 and M_2 than between M_3 and M_4. A hypothetical organization of metabolic system from these correlations is presented in Figure 3.13.

Interestingly, some positive correlations observed between concentrations corresponded to negative ones between relative levels; this concerns the pairs (M_1, M_3) and (M_2, M_3). Moreover, the negative correlation previously observed between concentrations of M_3 and M_4 showed a positive value when calculated on relative levels. By combining the negative and positive correlations observed with relative levels and concentrations, respectively, metabolite M_3 can be considered as belonging to a different pathway but sharing some biosynthetic factors with M_1 and M_2 (Figure 3.13).

More hypotheses on the origins of correlations in metabolomic datasets will be presented in the next section.

II.4. Interpretation of Origins of Correlations in Metabolic Systems

A high correlation between two metabolites can be originated from several mechanisms (Camacho et al. 2005):

1) Chemical equilibrium
2) Mass conservation
3) Assymetric control
4) Unusually high variance in the expression of a single gene

II.4.1. Chemical Equilibrium
Two metabolites near chemical equilibrium will show a high positive correlation, with a concentration ratio approximating the equilibrium constant. As a consequence, metabolites with negative correlation are *not* in equilibrium. Positive correlation can be observed between a precursor and its product having synchronous metabolic variations (Figure 3.14a).

II.4.2. Mass Conservation
Within a moiety-conserved cycle, at least one member should have a negative correlation with another member of the conserved group. This may be also the case for two metabolites competing for a same substrate (precursor) representing a limited source which has to be shared (Figure 3.14b-c).

II.4.3. Assymetric Control

Most high correlations may be due (a) to either strong mutual control by a single enzyme (Figure 3.14b), or (b) to variation of a single enzyme level much above others (Figure 3.14c). This may result from a metabolic pathway effect (Figure 3.14d): the variation of a single enzyme level within a metabolic pathway will have direct or indirect repercussions on the successive metabolites of such a pathway leading to their positive correlation(s). Such a positive correlation can be generally attributed to the shared effect(s) of common metabolic pathway that metabolites sustained against other pathways of the network. In the case where two metabolites are controlled by a same enzyme, the activity of such enzyme in favor to one metabolite at the expense of the other results in negative correlation between them; these two metabolites can belong to two different paths (e.g. M_1, M_5) or sub-paths (e.g. M_7, M_8). In more general terms, if one parameter dominates the concentration of two metabolites, intrinsic fluctuations of this parameter result in a high correlation between them.

Assymetric control can be graphically analysed by a log-log scatter plot between metabolites' concentrations (Camacho et al., 2005). From such a graphic, change in correlation reflects change in the co-response of the two metabolites toward the dominant parameter (Figure 3.15).

II.4.4. Unusually High Variance in the Expression of a Single Gene

This is similar to the previous situation but the resulting correlation is not due to a high sensitivity toward a particular parameter, but due to an unusually high variance of this parameter. In particular, a single enzyme that carries a high variance will induce negative correlations between its substrate and product metabolites (Steuer, 2006).

II.5. Scale-Dependent Interpretations of Correlations

The analysis of correlations exploits the intrinsic variability of a metabolic system to obtain additional features on the state of the system. The set of all the correlations (given by the correlation matrix) is a global property of the metabolic system, i.e. whether two metabolites are correlated or not does not depend solely on the reactions they participate in, but on the combined result of all the reactions and regulatory interactions present in the system. In this sense, the pattern of correlations between metabolites can be interpreted as a global fingerprint of the metabolic system at a given time integrating implicitly effects of environmental conditions, physiological states, etc.

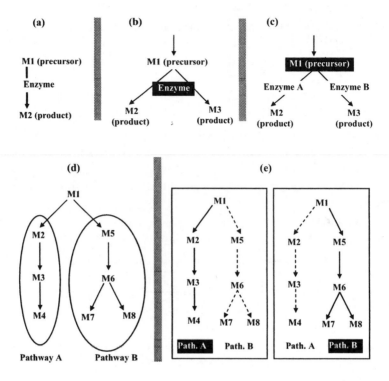

Figure 3.14. Different scales at which correlations between metabolites can be interpreted: metabolite (a-c), metabolic pathway (d), network (physiological)(e) scales.

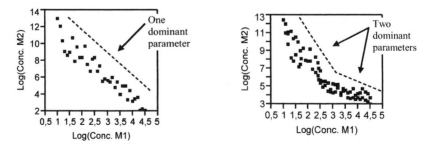

Figure 3.15. Some examples of Log-Log scatter plots used to detect co-response of two metabolites under the effect of some dominant parameter(s).

Apart from the variations due to temporal, physiological and environmental factors, the correlation between two metabolites can show scale-dependent variations within a same metabolic system: in a metabolic map, such variations are observed at local and global scales, providing evidence on the functional and topological complexity of metabolic system:

At a local scale, two metabolites are closely considered the one toward the other without consideration of the other metabolites. For example, two metabolites can be competitive for a same enzyme (Figure 3.14b) or a same precursor (Figure 3.14c) within a common metabolic pathway leading to a local negative correlation between them. However, a strongly synchronous variation between precursor and product leads to a positive local correlation.

At global scale, these two locally competitive metabolites are constituents of a same metabolic pathway which can compete other pathways (containing the other metabolites). The common metabolic pathway results in a positive global correlation between the two considered metabolites (Figure 3.14d: Metabolites M_7, M_8). The common metabolic pathway has a direct positive effect on these metabolites, because it results in shared biosynthesis factors and enzymatic regulation processes. Also, common metabolic pathway has indirect positive effect on the metabolites by the fact that it results in their shared competition against other metabolites belonging to other metabolic pathways (Figure 3.14d).

In summary, two metabolites can manifest global and local correlations with opposite signs, i.e. negative (positive) local and positive (negative) global correlations.

At metabolic map scale, there are many pairs of metabolites that are spatially neighbors but have low correlations, and others that are not neighbors but have high correlations. This is due to the fact that the correlations are shaped by both stoichiometric and kinetic effects (Steuer et al., 2003a, b).

At a higher scale, diminutive fluctuations within the metabolic system or in the environment conditions induce correlations which will propagate through the system to give rise to a specific pattern of correlations depending on the physiological state of the system (Camacho et al., 2005; Steuer et al., 2003a, b; Morgenthal et al., 2006) (Figure 3.14e).

A transition from a physiological state to another may not only involve changes in the average levels of the analysed metabolites but additionally may also involve changes in their correlations.

II.6. Multidimensional Correlation Screening by Means of Principle Component Analysis

II.6.1. Aim

Principle component analysis (PCA) is a multivariate analysis which uses the linear algebra rules to provide topological link between the n rows and p columns of a dataset (Waite, 2000). Using a minimum dimension space, PCA combines all information in dataset to calculate relative positions of row- and column-points which will be interpreted in terms of affinities, oppositions or independences between them; this helps to understand:

- specific characteristics of individuals (e.g. metabolic profiles) (row analysis),
- relative behaviors of variables (e.g. metabolites) (column analysis),
- associations between individuals and variables.

In the plan, row-points can show grouping into different "constellations" indicating the presence of different sub-populations in the dataset.

To topological analysis of rows and columns, PCA decomposes the variability space of a dataset into a succession of orthogonal axes representing decreasing and complementary parts of the total variability. From the simplistic illustration (Figure 3.16), decomposition of the total variability into two orthogonal directions F_1 and F_2 highlights clearly some similar and opposite behaviors of the different variables M_j : along F_1, the variables M_1 and M_2 show a certain affinity and seem to be opposite to the variables M_3 and M_4 (projected on the other extremity of F_1). Such information is completed by that along F_2 where M_1 and M_3 share a similar behavior opposite to that of the variables M_2 and M_4.

Taking into account the fact the first axis F_1 covers a higher variability than the second one F_2 (and so on), the affinities between M_1 and M_2 or M_3 and M_4 (along F_1) are stronger than those between M_1 and M_3 or M_2 and M_4 (along F_2).

This illustrates the aim of PCA consisting in handling the complex variability under successive complementary view angles.

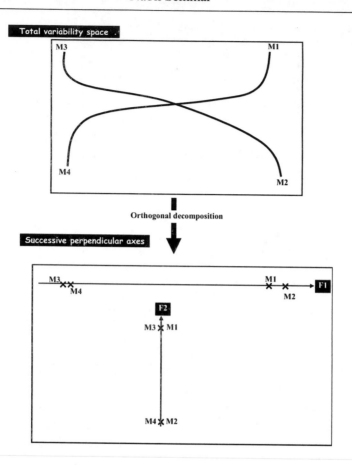

Figure 3.16. Simplistic illustration of decomposition of the total variability into additive (complementary) parts along perpendicular axes (F1, F2).

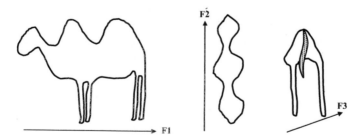

Figure 3.17. Intuitive illustration of the usefulness of orthogonal decomposition to describe a complex variability system through decreasing complementary parts (along F_k).

II.6.2. General principle of PCA

PCA is a decomposition approach based on the extraction of the eigenvalues and eigenvectors of a dataset. The eigenvectors, perpendicular between them, represent the bases of orthogonal directions called principle components (PCs) (F_k). The PCs extract complementary and decreasing parts of the total variability of a whole dataset (Figure 3.17).

The decreasing variability parts are closely linked to the eigenvalues sorted by decreasing order: to each eigenvalue λ_k of the dataset corresponds an eigenvector U_k the direction of which defines the principle component F_k; the variability covered by F_k is equal to λ_k and can be expressed in terms of relative part by $\lambda_k/\Sigma(\lambda_k)$ (Figure 3.18) (Waite, 2000).

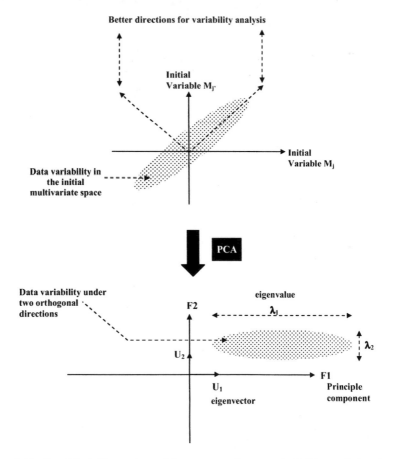

Figure 3.18. Graphical illustration of three successive steps in PCA consisting in calculating eigenvalues λ_k, eigenvectors U_k and principle components F_k

II.6.3. Computation of Eigenvalues, Eigenvectors and Principle Components

Eigenvalues and eigenvectors are calculated from a square $(p \times p)$ and invertible (not null determinant) matrix A. Under reversibility condition, the square matrix A $(p \times p)$ can be decomposed into p directions F_k defined by p eigenvectors U_k and weighted by p eigenvalues λ_k. From an experimental dataset X, a square matrix A can be directly obtained by the product $A = X'X$ where X' is the transpose of X; therefore, the eigenvalues and eigenvectors are calculated from A.

The eigenvalues λ_k and their corresponding eigenvectors U_k are extracted from the square matrix A $(p \times p)$ by solving the following matricial equation:

$$A.U = \lambda.U \Leftrightarrow A.U - \lambda.U = 0 \Leftrightarrow (A - \lambda.I). U = 0 \Leftrightarrow (A - \lambda.I) = 0 \quad (3.6)$$

$$\text{where I is a } (p \times p) \text{ identity matrix: } I = \begin{pmatrix} 1 & 0 & \cdots & 0 & 0 \\ 0 & 1 & \cdots & 0 & 0 \\ \cdots & \cdots & \cdots & \cdots & \cdots \\ 0 & 0 & \cdots & 1 & 0 \\ 0 & 0 & \cdots & 0 & 1 \end{pmatrix} \begin{matrix} 1 \\ \cdot \\ \cdot \\ \cdot \\ p \end{matrix}$$
$$\begin{matrix} 1 & \cdots & \cdots & \cdots & p \end{matrix}$$

This matricial equation is solved by setting its determinant to zero: $\det(A - \lambda.I) = 0$, leading to solve a p equations system with p unknowns λ_k. After computation of the eigenvalues λ_k, the corresponding eigenvectors U_k are calculated from the initial equation $A.U = \lambda.U$.

Finally, from the eigenvectors U_k, the initial variables M_j of the dataset X are replaced by "synthetic" variables F_k (called principle components) obtained by linear combinations of the p initial variables M_j affected by corresponding coordinates u_{jk} in the eigenvectors U_k:

$$F_{ik} = \sum_{j=1}^{p} X_{ij}U_{jk} = x_{i1}.u_{1k} + x_{i2}.u_{2k} + x_{i3}.u_{3k} + \ldots + x_{ij}.u_{jk} + \ldots + x_{ip}.u_{pk} \quad (3.7)$$

In other words, from the p coordinates x_{ij} of a row i corresponding to the p columns j ($j=1$ to p), a single new coordinate F_{ik} is calculated by Eq. 3.7 to represent the new position of row i along the principle component F_k (Figure 3.19). The n new coordinates, called factorial coordinates, provide condensed information on the behaviors of the n individuals i taking into account all the variables j at once along a high variability direction F_k. On this basis, the factorial coordinates are more appropriate to associate the different behaviors of individuals i to different levels of variables M_j, leading to understand different variability sources in the initial dataset X.

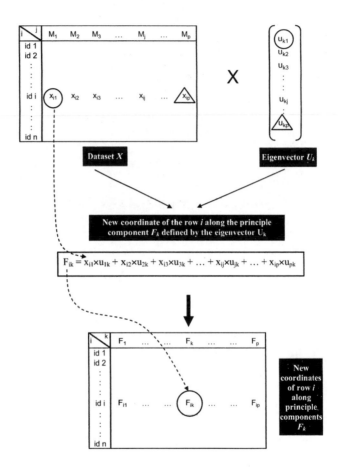

Figure 3.19. Computation of new coordinates (factorial coordinates) of an individuals i along a principle component F_k by a linear combination of its initial coordinates x_{ij} affected by the coordinates u_{jk} of the eigenvector U_k

To understand more the calculation and the interpretation of eigenvalues, eigenvectors and factorial coordinates in PCA, let's give a simplistic numerical example based on a square matrix A (2×2).

$$A = \begin{bmatrix} 2 & 3 \\ 3 & -6 \end{bmatrix}$$

$$A - \lambda.I = \begin{bmatrix} 2 & 3 \\ 3 & -6 \end{bmatrix} - \lambda \begin{bmatrix} 1 & 0 \\ 0 & 1 \end{bmatrix} = \begin{bmatrix} 2 & 3 \\ 3 & -6 \end{bmatrix} \begin{bmatrix} \lambda & 0 \\ 0 & \lambda \end{bmatrix} = \begin{bmatrix} 2 - \lambda & 3 \\ 3 & -6 - \lambda \end{bmatrix}$$

$$\det (A - \lambda.I) = \det \begin{bmatrix} 2 - \lambda & 3 \\ 3 & -6 - \lambda \end{bmatrix} \longrightarrow \det \begin{bmatrix} a & c \\ b & d \end{bmatrix} = ad - bc$$

$$\det \begin{bmatrix} 2 - \lambda & 3 \\ 3 & -6 - \lambda \end{bmatrix} = [(2 - \lambda)(-6 - \lambda) - 9] = \lambda^2 + 4\lambda - 21$$

Setting $\lambda^2 + 4\lambda - 21$ to 0 leads to the equivalent form: $(\lambda - 3)(\lambda + 7) = 0$, so the eigenvalues λ_k of A are 3 and -7. After sorting these two λ_k by decreasing absolute value, we have $\lambda_1 = -7$ and $\lambda_2 = 3$.

For each eigenvalue λ_k, the corresponding eigenvector U_k is calculated by solving the matricial equation $(A - \lambda.I).U = 0$:

For $\lambda_1 = -7$, the matricial equation will be:

$$\left(\begin{bmatrix} 2 & 3 \\ 3 & -6 \end{bmatrix} - (-7) \begin{bmatrix} 1 & 0 \\ 0 & 1 \end{bmatrix} \right) \begin{bmatrix} u_{11} \\ u_{21} \end{bmatrix} = 0 \quad \Leftrightarrow \quad \left(\begin{bmatrix} 2 & 3 \\ 3 & -6 \end{bmatrix} + \begin{bmatrix} 7 & 0 \\ 0 & 7 \end{bmatrix} \right) \begin{bmatrix} u_{11} \\ u_{21} \end{bmatrix} = 0$$

$$\Leftrightarrow \begin{bmatrix} 9 & 3 \\ 3 & 1 \end{bmatrix} \begin{bmatrix} u_{11} \\ u_{21} \end{bmatrix} = 0$$

This leads to the following equation system:

$$\begin{array}{lll} 9u_{11} + 3u_{21} = 0 & \Leftrightarrow & 9u_{11} = -3u_{21} \\ 3u_{11} + u_{21} = 0 & \Leftrightarrow & 3u_{11} = -u_{21} \end{array} \Bigg\} \Leftrightarrow 3u_{11} = -u_{21}$$

For $u_{11} = 1$, we have $u_{21} = -3$. Therefore, $U_1 = (1, -3)$ represents the first eigenvector of A.

Note that due to the fact that the equation system is reduced to one equation with two unknown, results in the existence of infinity of eigenvectors proportional to U_1.

For $\lambda_2 = 3$, the matricial equation will be:

$$\left(\begin{bmatrix} 2 & 3 \\ 3 & -6 \end{bmatrix} - (3)\begin{bmatrix} 1 & 0 \\ 0 & 1 \end{bmatrix}\right)\begin{bmatrix} u_{12} \\ u_{22} \end{bmatrix} = 0 \qquad \Leftrightarrow \left(\begin{bmatrix} 2 & 3 \\ 3 & -6 \end{bmatrix} - \begin{bmatrix} 3 & 0 \\ 0 & 3 \end{bmatrix}\right)\begin{bmatrix} u_{12} \\ u_{22} \end{bmatrix} = 0$$

$$\Leftrightarrow \begin{bmatrix} -1 & 3 \\ 3 & -9 \end{bmatrix}\begin{bmatrix} u_{12} \\ u_{22} \end{bmatrix} = 0$$

This leads to the following equation system:

$$\begin{array}{ll} -u_{12} + 3u_{22} = 0 & \Leftrightarrow \quad u_{12} = 3u_{22} \\ 3u_{12} - 9u_{22} = 0 & \Leftrightarrow \quad 3u_{12} = 9u_{22} \end{array} \Bigg\} \Leftrightarrow u_{12} = 3u_{22}$$

For $u_{22} = 1$, we have $u_{12} = 3$. Therefore, $U_2 = (3, 1)$ represents the second eigenvector of A.

Also, the fact that the equation system is reduced to one equation with two unknown results in the existence of infinity of eigenvectors proportional to U_2.

The two calculated eigenvectors U_1 and U_2 define a new basis of orthogonal directions along which the row and column variability of the dataset A can be topologically analysed (Figure 3.20).

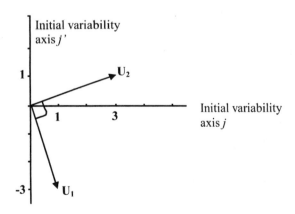

Figure 3.20. Illustration of the orthogonality between the eigenvectors of a square matrix.

After calculation of the eigenvectors U_1 and U_2, the new coordinates F_{ik} of the rows i along the principal components F_k (k=1 to 2) can be calculated by the scalar products $A.U_k$. Thus, along the principle component F_1 defined by the direction of U_1, the two rows of the matrix A will be represented by two coordinates given by:

$$A.U_1 = \begin{pmatrix} 2 & 3 \\ 3 & -6 \end{pmatrix} \begin{bmatrix} 1 \\ -3 \end{bmatrix} = \begin{bmatrix} -7 \\ 21 \end{bmatrix} ;$$ this result is also obtained by the product $\lambda_1.U_1$.

Along the second principle component F_2, each row of the matrix A will have a new coordinate given by:

$$A.U_2 = \begin{pmatrix} 2 & 3 \\ 3 & -6 \end{pmatrix} \begin{bmatrix} 3 \\ 1 \end{bmatrix} = \begin{bmatrix} 9 \\ 3 \end{bmatrix};$$ this result is also obtained by the product $\lambda_2.U_2$.

Finally, the dataset A can be replaced by the new matrix F giving the factorial coordinates of the individuals (rows) i along each principle component F_k (k=1, 2):

$$F = \begin{bmatrix} -7 & 9 \\ 21 & 3 \end{bmatrix}$$

From F, the individuals of the dataset A can be projected on the plane F_1F_2 for a topological analysis of their variability (Figure 3.21). To link the variability of individuals to that of variables, a variable plot can be obtained from the coordinates of the eigenvectors by which the initial variables were weighted (Figure 3.21). According to their absolute values, the eigenvectors' coordinates attribute more or less importance to the initial variables M_j in the new (factorial) coordinates of individuals i. For example, the individual id_1 has a factorial coordinate equal to -7 on F_1; this value was calculated by the following linear combination:

$$-7 = (id1).U1 = (2\ 3)\begin{bmatrix} 1 \\ -3 \end{bmatrix} = (2 \times 1) + (3 \times \boxed{-3}\ )$$

In this linear combination, the second variable M_2 is affected by an eigenvector score equal to -3 the absolute value of which (Abs(-3)=3) is higher than the coordinate=1 by which is affected the first variable M_1. This gives a higher weight of M_2 than M_1 along F_1. This helps to conclude that the variability of all the individuals on F_1 is mainly due to the variable M_2. Graphically, this can be showed by a projection of M_2 both at extremity and close to the axis F_1 (Figure 3.21). Moreover, the roles of variables M_j on the different principle components F_k can be evaluated by computing their absolute contributions in relation to their factorial coordinates and the eigenvalues. Contribution computation will be detailed in this chapter (§ II.8.2.7; Eq. 3.17).

II.6.4. Graphical Interpretation of Factorial Plans

According to the factorial plan F_1F_2 of individuals (Figure 3.21), id_1 and id_2 show opposition along F_1. According to the variable plot, the variables M_1 and M_2 seem to be opposite, and projected on the same sides than id_2 and id_1, respectively. Taking into account the importance of variable M_2 on F_1, the variability along F_1 can be mainly explained by M_2: thus, the graphical proximity between M_2 and id_1 and the opposition of id_1 to id_2 can be explained by a high value of M_2 in id_1 and a low one in id_2. In fact, in the initial dataset A, the values of M_2 are $+3$ and -6 in id_1 and id_2, respectively. Thus, PCA helped to identify that the highest variability source in the dataset A consisted of an important opposition between id_1 and id_2 for variable M_2. In metabolomic terms, this can correspond to a situation where some individuals are productive of a metabolite M_2 whereas others are relatively deficient in M_2.

For F_2, the highest coordinate of corresponding eigenvector U_2 concerns variable M_1, leading to deduce that the role of M_1 on F_2 is relatively more important than that of M_2. Graphically, the variable M_1 projects in the same side on F_2 than individuals id_1 and id_2, but it shows more proximity to id_2. This translates a higher value of M_1 in id_2 than in id_1; this can be checked in the initial dataset A. From this simplistic example, variable M_2 appears to play a separation role between individuals (profiles), whereas the variable M_1 seems to group the individuals according to a more or less high affinity. The fact that id_1 and id_2 are not opposite along F_2 can be attributed to their relatively close positive values (2 and 3, respectively).

Apart from the association analysis between rows (individuals) and columns (variables), the interpretations in PCA can be focused on the variability of variables and individuals, separately: on the plan F_1F_2 (Figure 3.21), the variables M_1 and M_2 seem to have mainly opposite behaviors from their projections in two different parts of the plan. This opposition is observed for individuals, and seems to indicate the presence of two trends in the initial dataset A. These two trends can be checked in the matrix A by opposite variations of M_1 and M_2 between id_1 and id_2.

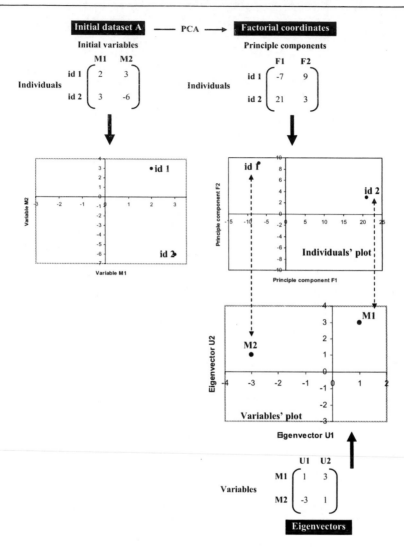

Figure 3.21. Graphical analysis based on principle component analysis (PCA) giving links between the variability of individuals and that of variables.

II.6.5. Different Types of PCA

The variability of a dataset X ($n \times p$) can be analysed by different types of PCA based on different criteria by considering (Figure 3.22):

-   Crude data leading to give more consideration to the most dispersed variables from the axes' origin.

- Data variations around their mean vector (centered PCA) leading to analyse the variability of the dataset around its gravity centre GC.
- Standardized data obtained by homogenizing the variation scales of all the variables through their weighting by their standard deviations. This leads to analyse the variability of the dataset within a unity scale space.
- Ranked data using the ranks of data rather than their values.

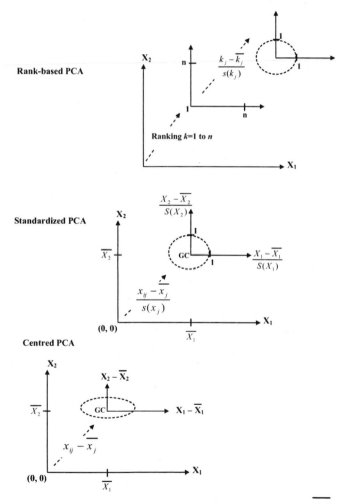

Figure 3.22. Illustration of different data transformations in PCA. X_j, $\overline{X}_j$, $S(X_j)$: data vector, mean and standard deviation of variable j, respectively. K_j: vector containing ranks of values of variable j. GC: gravity centre.

These different PCA are performed from diffe   square matrices ($p \times p$):

- PCA on crude data is performed on the square matrix $X'X$.
- Centered PCA is performed on the square matrix $C'C$, with $C = X - \overline{X}$, and where $\overline{X}$ is the mean vector of the different variables.
- Standardized PCA is applied on the square matrix $Z'Z$, with $Z = \dfrac{X - \overline{X}}{SD}$, and where $\overline{X}$ and SD are the mean and standard deviation of each corresponding variable, respectively.
- Rank-based PCA is applied on the square matrix $K'K$, where K is the rank matrix containing the data ranks for each variable of dataset X.

The applications of these different PCA require some conditions and have different interests:

Centered PCA can be applied when all the variables have the same unit (e.g. µg/ml). Its interest consists in highlighting the effect of the most dispersed variables on the structure of the dataset. Thus, the most dispersed variables can be considered as more rich in information than the less dispersed ones. Centered PCA helps to identify how the individuals (profiles) are separated the ones from the others under the dispersion effect of some variables. Moreover, centered PCA allows separation of the different variables according to their variation scales and directions (i.e. according to their covariances). In centered PCA, the sum of the eigenvalues is equal to the total variance of the dataset.

Standardized PCA is required when the dataset consists of heterogeneous variables expressed with different measure units (µg, ml, °c, etc.). Also, it is required when the variables (with same measure unit) have different variation scales due to incomparable variances (heteroscedasticity). In these cases, the values of each variable X_j are standardized by subtracting the mean $\overline{X}_j$ and by dividing by the standard deviation SD_j. The standardizations are appropriate preliminary transformations to analyse correlations between variables. The linear combination calculus on standardized data attributes to the variables relative positions which are graphically interpretable in terms of Pearson correlations: on factorial plans of PCA, the co-response of two variables will be highlighted by two vectors which will be projected along a same direction of the multivariate space. The correlation between two variables is graphically given by the cosine of their corresponding vectors. If two variables are positively correlated, their corresponding vectors will have a very sharp angle

($0\leq \leq\pi/4$) (positive cosine); in the case of negatively correlated variables, the corresponding vectors will be opposite, i.e. their angle will be strongly obtuse ($3\pi/4\leq \leq\pi$) (negative cosine). In the case of low correlations, the two vectors corresponding to the paired variables will have almost perpendicular directions. In standardized PCA, the sum of the eigenvalues is equal to the number (p) of variables.

Rank-based PCA finds an exclusive application on ordinal qualitative dataset where the variables are not measured but consist of different classification modalities of the individuals (e.g. modalities low, intermediate, high levels). After substitution of the ordinal data by their ranks, a standardized PCA can be applied to analyse correlations between the qualitative variables on the basis of Spearman statistics. Rank-based PCA finds also application on heterogeneous continuous datasets because of different variable units or because of imbalanced variation ranges of the variables. In this sense, ranked PCA can provide an alternative way to the classic standardized PCA

II.6.6. Numerical Application and Interpretation of Standardized PCA

The application of standardized PCA will be illustrated by a numerical example based on a dataset of $n=9$ rows and $p=5$ columns (Figure 3.23). Under a metabolomic aspect, let's consider the rows as metabolic profiles, the columns as metabolites and the continuous data as concentrations.

The PCA gives two principle components F_1 and F_2 associated to two eigenvalues $\lambda_1=3.74$ and $\lambda_2=1.20$. Such eigenvalues correspond to 75% ($3.74/p$) and 24% ($1.20/p$) of the total variability extracted by F_1 and F_2, respectively.

On the plot of individuals, the nine points are projected according to three trends (Figure 3.23): $id_{1, 2, 3}$ (group G1), $id_{4, 5, 6}$ (group G2) and $id_{7, 8, 9}$ (group G3). Groups G1 and G2 are opposite along the first component F_1; this means that they have opposite characteristics: according to the correlation circle, the variable M_3 projects closely to the individuals of G1, meaning that its values are high in these individuals. On this basis, the graphical proximity between variables M_1, M_4, M_5 and individuals $id_{4, 5, 6}$ leads to conclude that the group G2 is characterized by high values for these variables. Finally, the variable M_2 projects in a part where no individual is concerned. However, it appears to be opposite to G1 along F_1 and to G3 (particularly) along F_2. This means that the variable M_2 is an opposition variable characterizing individuals by low values: in fact the individuals id_1, id_2 and id_7-id_9 have relatively low values for M_2, whereas id_5, id_6 (graphically closer to M_2) showed relatively higher values for M_2 (Figure 3.23).

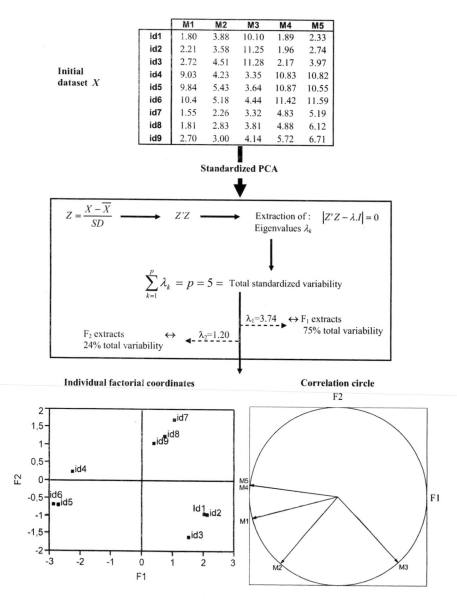

Figure 3.23. Graphical representations of a standardized PCA based on the factorial coordinates' plot of individuals and correlation circle of variables. X, $\overline{X}$, SD: data, means and standard deviations of different variables M_j, respectively.

From the correlation circle, affinity and opposition between the variables can be highlighted from sharp or obtuse angles between corresponding vectors: thus, the vectors M_4, M_5 and M_1 show very sharp angles meaning positive correlations between corresponding variables (Figure 3.24). On the other hand, the vector of M_3 seems to be particularly opposite to those of M_4, M_5 meaning negative correlations between their corresponding variables. M_1 and M_3 have almost perpendicular obtuse vectors (Figure 3.23) meaning a low or not significant correlation between them (Figure 3.24). The vectors M_2 and M_3 are closer to the orthogonality than (M_1, M_3), and represent a stronger independence state between corresponding variables. Finally, the vector M_2 shares a sharp angle with M_1 and in a lesser measure with M_4 and M_5. This means a positive correlation of variable M_2 toward M_1, which is higher than those toward M_4 and M_5.

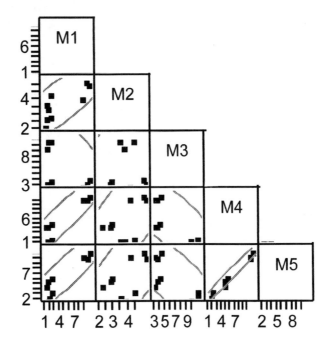

Figure 3.24. Scatter plot matrix showing the correlations between different variables M_1-M_5 projected on correlation circle of standardized PCA presented in figure 3.23. High correlations are indicated by thin confidence ellipses.

II.7. Metabolic Control Analysis

II.7.1. General Principle and Aim

Metabolic control analysis (MCA) aims at understanding the control each step of a given metabolic pathway exerts on system variables (flux, concentration). It is basically a sensitivity analysis of metabolic system which brings conceptual and mathematical formalisms of the relative contributions of individual effectors in a metabolic pathway to both the flux and the concentrations of intermediates within the pathway. Thus, by quantifying control processes of metabolic flux, MCA represents a powerful tool for describing and analysing the theoretical aspects of metabolic regulation (Kacser and Burns, 1973).

MCA is a sensitivity analysis applied to a steady state network system which submits small perturbations. Such perturbations exert influence both directly by local (system compartments) changes and indirectly by modulations of surrounding fluxes and concentrations at global (whole system) level. Analysis of metabolic responses resulting from such small perturbations provide information on different control processes and limiting steps at different scales of metabolic system: at local scale, MCA assesses the systemic relevance of a specific enzyme activity on a particular flux; at global scale, MCA helps to quantify how the distributions of SS fluxes and concentrations are controlled through different the reactions/steps of metabolic network.

MCA is a kinetic approach because it integrates local kinetic information (enzymatic kinetics) to quantify proportions of control exerted by different components of a given pathway or subsystem. This helps to identify the kinetic constraints in a biochemical network leading to determine the rate-limiting reaction in the system (Kacser and Burns, 1973; Heinrich et al., 1997).

Under experimental aspect, MCA explores unknown metabolic systems through two ways: (1) flux is changed and impact on the levels of the direct and indirect products of gene action is measured. (2) The levels of individual gene products are altered, and the impact on the flux is measured (Castrillo et al., 2007).

Under computational aspect, the system sensitivity is analysed from system response to an external perturbation using partitionned response coefficients. The system perturbation can be analysed from a collection of metabolic concentration measurements obtained from multiple observations of replicate biological samples: the variance observed in these measurements can be considered to arise from slight differences in internal and/or external parameters between samples, such as enzyme concentrations, kinetic constraints and environmental conditions.

Finally, the results given by MCA can be useful for correlation analysis because the different response coefficients provide information on mutual behaviors/responses of different system variables leading to interpret correlations between such variables (e.g. metabolites) (Camacho et al., 2005).

II.7.2. Principles and Methodology of MCA

Being a sensitivity analysis, MCA uses normalized sensitivity measures to quantify how the control of steady state fluxes and concentrations is distributed between different reactions in a metabolic network. The normalized sensitivity measures include two coefficient types: control and elasticity coefficients.

Control coefficient can define the degree of control that each step in a pathway has on the system. Among control coefficients, flux control and concentration control coefficients measure the degree of control exerted by enzyme (the control parameter) on flux and metabolite concentrations, respectively. Mathematically, the sensitivity of a state parameter X_i toward the change in a control parameter p_k can be formulated by means of the response or control coefficient $R_{p_k}^{X_i}$ (Eq. 3.8) (Yang et al., 1998; Wildermuth, 2000; Moreno-Sánchez, 2008):

$$R_{p_k}^{X_i} = \frac{\dfrac{dX_i}{X_i^0}}{\dfrac{dp_k}{p_k^0}} = \frac{d \ln X_i}{d \ln p_k} \tag{3.8}$$

Where:

X_i: value of state parameter i (e.g. flux or concentration of interest)

X_i^0: reference value of state parameter i

P_k: value of control parameter k that changed (e.g. enzyme concentration)

p_k^0: reference value of considered control parameter k

The dimensionless control coefficient $R_{p_k}^{X_i}$ represents a proportionality constant to calculate the displacement ($\Delta \ln X_i$) of state parameter from the knowledge of control parameter change ($\Delta \ln p_k$):

$$\Delta \ln X_i = R_{p_k}^{X_i} \Delta \ln p_k \qquad (3.9)$$

However, such a proportionality relationship between state variables (flux, substrate or metabolite concentration) and control parameter (e.g. enzyme concentration) is an approximation because the responses are generally non-linear.

The case of single control parameter expressed by equation (3.9) can be generalized to q parameters by writing the displacement of state variable as a sum of q terms, each one corresponding to the effect of a single parameter:

$$\Delta \ln X_i = \sum_{k=1}^{q} R_{p_k}^{X_i} \Delta \ln p_k \qquad (3.10)$$

When two metabolites X_i and $X_{i'}$ suffer from multiple perturbations (due to q parameters p_k), their relative variations resulting from the global effect of all the parameters can be estimated by the ratio of their displacements, i.e. the ratio of the sums of products between the q parameters p_k and control coefficients $R_{p_k}^{X}$:

$$\frac{\Delta \ln X_i}{\Delta \ln X_{i'}} \approx \frac{\displaystyle\sum_{k=1}^{q} R_{p_k}^{X_i} \Delta \ln p_k}{\displaystyle\sum_{k=1}^{q} R_{p_k}^{X_{i'}} \Delta \ln p_k} \qquad (3.11)$$

The use of flux or concentration as system state parameters results in the defintion of two control coefficients consisting of flux control (FCC or $R_{p_k}^{v_j}$) and concentration control coefficients (CCC or $R_{p_k}^{C_i}$), respectively (Eqs. 3.11, 3.12):

$$FCC = R_{p_k}^{v_j} = \frac{d \ln v_j}{d \ln p_k} \qquad (3.12)$$

$$CCC = R_{p_k}^{C_i} = \frac{d \ln C_i}{d \ln p_k}$$ (3.13)

Where:

v_j: flux of chemical reaction j
C_i: concentration of metabolite i
p_k: value of control parameter k

FCC and CCC quantify the normalized changes in the steady state level of flux and biochemical concentration, respectively, in response to a relative change in control parameter (e.g. normalized concentration of catalyzing enzyme) (Kacser and Burns, 1973; Heinrich and Rapoport, 1974).

Elasticity coefficient (or the elasticity) $\varepsilon_{X_i}^{v_j}$ is a dimensionless measure of the fractional change in a reaction rate v_j upon changes in the concentration X_i of a ligand (substrate, product, allosteric modulator) (Rodríguez-Enríquez et al., 2000; Zu and Guppy, 2004; Erecinska and Dagani, 1990; Brown et al., 1990; Hafner et al., 1990; Wanders et al., 1984; Groen et al., 1986; Marín-Hernández et al., 2006; Kruckeberg et al., 1989):

$$\varepsilon_{X_i}^{v_j} = \frac{\dfrac{dv_j}{v_j^0}}{\dfrac{dX_i}{X_i^0}} = \frac{d \ln v_j}{d \ln X_i}$$ (3.14)

Where:

v_j^0 : reference value of reaction rate v_j

X_i^0 : reference concentration value of ligand X_i

Elasticity coefficient can be positive, negative or close to zero. It is:
-   Positive for metabolites that increase the enzyme or transporter rate v_j. This can be checked for substrates or activators.
-   Negative for metabolites that decrease the enzyme or transporter rates (final produts or inhibitors)

- Null or close to zero for an enzyme working under a steady state metabolic flux, at saturing conditions of substrate or product. Under such conditions, the enyme is no longer sensitive to changes in these metabolites.

However, an enzyme working at substrate (S) or product (P) concentrations lower than the Michaelis constant (Km_s or Km_p) is expected to be highly sensitive to small variations in S or P (Figure 3.25).

The elasticities are intrinsically linked to the actual enzyme kinetics: if the kinetic parameters of an enzyme are known (Vm, Km), the enzyme elasticity to a given metabolite concentration can be calculated.

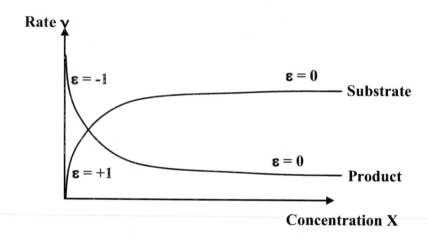

Figure 3.25. Variation in the values and signs of elasticity coefficient ε associated to different sensitivities of enzyme rate toward substrate or product concentration X.

II.7.3. Interpretation of MCA Results in Terms of Correlations

When the concentrations of two metabolites X_i and $X_{i'}$ are strictly perturbed by a same and unique parameter p_k (dominant parameter), the ratio of their control coefficients $R_{p_k}^{X_i}$ and $R_{p_k}^{X_{i'}}$ can be reduced to a constant $^{P_k}O_{X_{i'}}^{X_i}$ called co-response coefficient (Hofmeyr and Cornish-Bowden, 1996; Hofmeyr et al., 1993). Thus for a well defined dominant parameter p_k, the co-response coefficient $^{P_k}O_{X_{i'}}^{X_i}$ of two metabolites' concentrations X_i and $X_{i'}$ can be calculated by:

$$\frac{\Delta \ln X_i}{\Delta \ln X_{i'}} \approx \frac{R_{p_k}^{X_i} \Delta \ln p_k}{R_{p_k}^{X_{i'}} \Delta \ln p_k} = \frac{R_{p_k}^{X_i}}{R_{p_k}^{X_{i'}}} = {}^{p_k}O_{X_{i'}}^{X_i} \qquad (3.15)$$

This special case can occur when:

- The variability of one control parameter is much higher than that of any other parameter.
- The response of the two concentrations towards one control parameter are much higher than towards any other.

In these circumstances, the contribution of one parameter on the concentrations of the two metabolites dominates, and the other parameters become negligible. This situation is compatible with a high correlation coefficient between the concentrations X_i and $X_{i'}$ of the two metabolites i and i'.

Graphically, the scatter plot of $\ln(X_{i'})$ vs $\ln(X_i)$ obtained under the variations of the q parameters at once will correspond to a stretched shape cloud, i.e. a lines-like shape. The slope α of such a line is equal to the co-response coefficient, and consequently the correlation will be high. Positive slope can be interpreted as two metabolites in (or close to) chemical equilibrium. Negative slope indicates two metabolites varying each at expense of the other under the constraint of mass conservation (Hofmeyr et al., 1986).

Such correlation interpretation is valid however only under linearity conditions. Therefore, the linearity field must be determined and checked from replicates of biological samples which can represent either (i) a single or (ii) two (or more) physiological states:

i) Response coefficients are linear approximations around a reference state, but biochemical systems are governed by non-linear interactions. Therefore, it is important to determine the conditions and the variation range under which the studied physiological system could be linearly approximated.

ii) Replicated samples issued from two physiological states can be used to compare the scatter plots representing separately such states. This will be particularly important when in one physiological state, there is a high correlation, but not in the other (Figure 3.26a), or when the correlations are both high but of opposite signs (Figure 3.26b).

Finally, one should be careful to avoid false interpretations due to artefactual correlations. This could occur when:

- Two different physiological states give a single scatter plot with low correlation whereas high correlations are detected under each state alone (Figure 3.26c).
- The mean values of the concentrations of the two physiological states differ by a large amount resulting in a scatter plot with two separated clusters and leading to a spurious high correlation. This will happen even if no correlation exist in each separated state (Figure 3.26d).

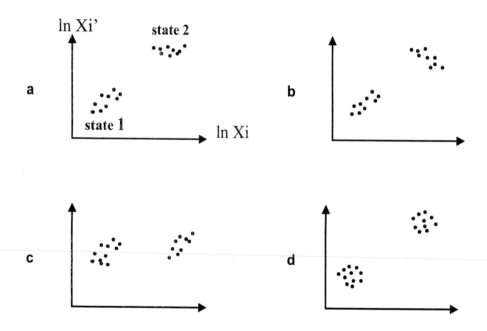

Figure 3.26. Graphical illustrations of different cases of physiological state-dependent correlations between metabolite concentrations X_i and $X_{i'}$ leading to interpret carefully co-response coefficient of the two metabolites i and i'.

Apart from correltions between metabolites, correlations between metabolic responses and external control factors can be assessed by means of MCA:

If FCC are known, relative priority for genetic modifications can be reached accordingly, since a high value suggests a large impact upon a reengineered enzyme activity.

Moreover, the FCC of any enzyme can be used to indirectly correlate metabolic responses with control environmental factors, because FCC is not constant, but rather a system property varying with environmental conditions.

II.8. Regression Analysis based on latent variables

II.8.1. General Principle and Aim

Latent variables can be defined as non directly measurable variables which are built by combining a mass of information issued from experimental data. Such intermediate variables are powerfull indicators issued from different computational methods. Principle components calculated in PCA are an example of latent variables. Latent variables can be used to build models helping to approach complex systems or complex concepts (e.g. intelligence, life state, anxiety, various interactions within and between biological systems, etc.). In biological system analysis, latent variables can be particularly useful to statistically explore links between different functional moities of a whole complex system. An illustrative example consists in searching relationships between metabolic responses and genetic variables combined with environmental factors. In terms of experimental data, these three fields of whole biological system are generally described by different types of variables:

Genetic data consist generally of a set of genes characterized by presences-absences in different biological organisms. Statistically, the different genes can be considered as binary qualitative variables because their presences or absences represent two mutually exclusive possibilities in all the individuals of biological population. Environmental conditions include generally various types of variables (continue as temperature, discrete as counting, qualitative as geographical origin). Metabolic data are generally represented by concentrations (continue variables) of different metabolites produced by the different individuals of the studied population. Such data are known to be continue.

Combining these different types of datasets, each individual is initially characterized by qualitative and quantitative variables representing its genetics, environmental conditions and metabolic system. Therefore, it becomes interesting to analyse correlations between metabolism and genetics under different environmental conditions. This can be expressed by different questions:

-   How the genetic profile can influence the metabolism taking into
    account external (stimulating/repressing) factors?
-   In the genetic profile, what gene(s) is (are) the most influent on such
    or such metabolite(s) regulation(s)?
-   Is it possible to predict the quantitative variations of a given
    metabolite from the variability of genetic profiles containing genes
    playing key roles in such a metabolism?

These questions can find responses by developing a statistical model
which has to predict continue data (concentrations) from qualitative profiles
which can include genetics, sex, environment type, etc. (Figure 3.27a). For
that, the qualitative descriptive data must be transformed into continue type,
then the resulting latent (continue) variables will be used to develop a
predictive regression model estimating the concentrations.

From the predictive regression model, the most influent (significant) latent
variables will be identified leading to a simplification of the final model. Their
interpretations in terms of initial qualitative variables (e.g. genetics, sex,
environment type, etc.) can be based on a sensitivity analysis taking into
account the contributions of the initial variables to the intermediate latent ones.
Finally, the predictive model needs to be validated on external data which
were not used in its building.

II.8.2. Methodology

II.8.2.1. Data Transformation Requirement

To develop a regression model predicting a continue variable (e.g.
metabolite concentration) from qualitative profile (e.g. genetic binary data),
two successive data transformations are needed (Figure 3.27):

-   After encoding of different qualitative variables into binary type
    (Figure 3.27b), the first transformation aims at conversion of the
    binary data (1, 0) to relative values by reference to both rows' and
    columns' sums of the binary dataset. Such qualitative data
    transformation can be obtained by applying a correspondence analysis
    (CA) leading to replace 0 and 1 by their factorial (continue)
    coordinates (Figure 3.27c). The principle and application of CA are
    illustrated in chapter 5 (§ VI.3). This CA-based data transformation is
    necessary to convert binary information into continue type, but it is
    not sufficient to develop a regression model predicting concentrations

from genetic data: the reason is that CA gives continue factorial coordinates which are distributed within a Chi-2 metric space, whereas the concentrations are continue data distributed within Euclidean-metric space.

- Therefore, it becomes necessary to carry out a second transformation type by which the factorial coordinates associated to Chi-2 metric will be converted into continue data associated to the Euclidean metric. Such a final conversion can be obtained by means of a standardized PCA applied on the factorial coordinates of CA (Figure 3.27d).
- Finally, PCA gives new factorial coordinates varying in Euclidean space which can be used to build a predictive regression model of concentrations from transformed qualitative data (Figure 3.27e). Such a model needs to be validated on an outside dataset, then its results can be interpreted after a sensitivity analysis.

This predictive approach of a continue variable from binary profiles will be illustrated by a numerical example presented in figures 3.30 and 3.31. Also, its different steps will be detailed in the next sections (Figures 3.27-3.29).

II.8.2.2. Binary encoding of qualitative variables

Starting from a dataset of qualitative characteristics (columns) in n individuals (n rows), binary codes 1 and 0 can be used to represent the presences and absences of such characteristics in such individuals (Escofier and Pages, 1991). There are two techniques to encode qualitative characteristics by binary data:

- For a given qualitative variable, its modalities will be represented by separated exclusive columns; then one puts 1 in the column of observed modality and 0 in the remaining (excluded) modality columns (Figure 3.28a). This encoding using as much columns as modalities, represents a general procedure and it is used when a qualitative variable has more than two modalities (e.g. geographical sites: S1, S2, S3; colors: blue, red, green, etc).
- In the case where a qualitative variable has only two exclusive modalities (e.g. sex), the code 1 can be used for one modality leading to use 0 for the other. In this case, the totality of information of the qualitative variable can be condensed into a single binary column containing 1 for a modality and 0 for the other modality (Figure 3.28b; 3.27b). In such cases, one modality will be represented by the

value 1 and the other by 0. Such a condensed encoding expects results directly interpretable by reference to the presence of the first modality, and indirectly by reference to the presence of the second modality which is synonym of the absence of the first one.

After encoding of all the qualitative characteristics into binary variables, one obtains a binary table with p columns, called disjonctive table D (Figure 3.27b). When, all the modalities are represented in distinct columns, the resulting binary table is called complete disjonctive table (Figure 3.28a).

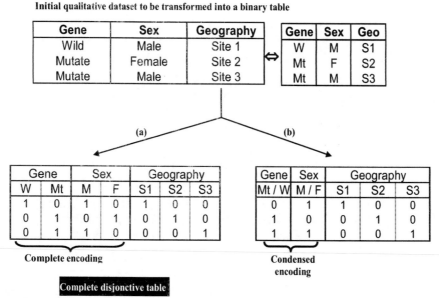

Figure 3.28. Two ways to binary encoding of a qualitative dataset. (a) Complete and (b) condensed encodings.

II.8.2.3. Correspondence Analysis
on Binary Dataset

From the disjonctive table D (n rows $\times p$ columns), a CA can be applied to analyse the relative states of all the binary values 1 and 0 by reference to the sums of both their rows and columns (Figure 3.29a).

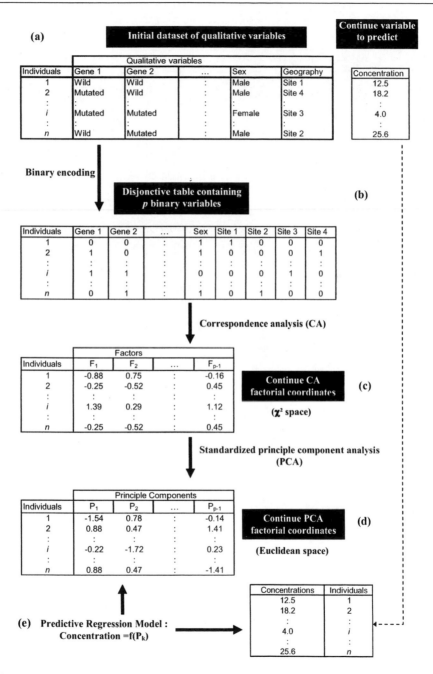

Figure 3.27. Successive transformations "CA-PCA" converting binary data to continue data associated to Euclidean metric ready to be used in a predictive regression model of concentrations.

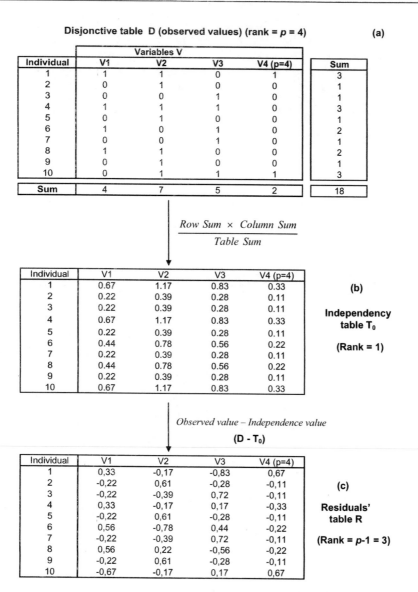

Figure 3.29. Numerical example illustrating the calculation of residuals' table from a disjonctive matrix. Residuals' table contains information on relative state of each qualitative variable in each individual by reference to a neutral state defined by the χ^2-independence criterion.

For that, CA considers the binary values by reference to their corresponding theoretical values calculated by the χ^2-independence rule

(Figure 3.29b): independence values are calculated from the products of sums of rows by sums of columns divided by the constant sum of the disjonctive table.

Disjonctive table D (n rows $\times$ p columns) has a rank equal to its lowest dimension, which corresponds generally to p ($p \ll n$ in general). However, the independence table T_0 issued directly from products of marginal sums divided by the constant sum of D has a rank equal to 1 (Figure 3.29b). Therefore, from the p-rank matrix D and the 1-rank independence matrix T_0, a residual table R (with rank = p-1) will be calculated by the subtraction R = D $-$ T_0 (Figure 3.29c). Residual matrix R contains interesting information around the question of how much each binary value (0 or 1) of D is close or far from the independence or neutrality frequency represented by T_0: for a given individual and a given variable, a higher absolute value of residual indicates a situation which is more far from the independence. Consequently, an individual (id) having a high residual for a variable can be considered as well differentiated by such a binary variable in the whole population. For example in figure 3.29c, id1 has a high absolute value for residuals of variables V_3 (0.83) and V_4 (0.67): by returning to the initial binary dataset, id1 can be characterized by V_3 because it is the only individual having a 0 for V_3 in presence of 1 for all the other variables. Moreover, id1 is characterized by V_4 because the value 1 of V_4 is rare (two individuals have 1 among ten). Inversely, a residual value close to zero indicates indifference (or small association) between the individual and the qualitative variable. Such original information can be extracted, structured and condensed by CA which will be used to transform the binary table D into continue type data:

From the matrix D (p-rank), CA extracts p-1 eigenvectors associated to (p-1) eigenvalues then it calculates p-1 factorial coordinates for each individual along the directions defined by the p-1 eigenvectors. Details and illustrations on the methodology of CA can be consulted in chapter 5 (Figures 5.12-5.14). From the numerical example of figure 3.30a, application of CA on a disjonctive table with p=4 binary variables leads to replace D by a factorial coordinate matrix containing p-1=3 columns (called factors F_1-F_3) and associated to 3 eigenvectors U_1-U_3 (initially calculated) (Figure 3.30b).

II.8.2.4. Transformation of Continue Data
from Chi-2 Space to Euclidean Space

CA will represent the n rows (individuals) of the matrix D in IR^{p-1}, i.e. n row vectors with p-1 coordinates. By the fact that the values are considered by reference to the sums of their rows and columns, the n profiles of (p-1) factorial coordinates will be distributed into a $(p-1)$-dimensions space associated to a Chi-2 metric.

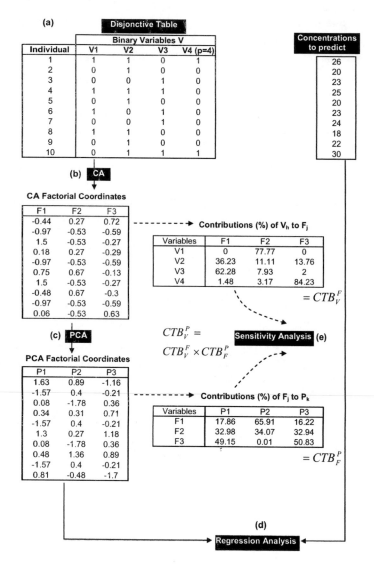

Figure 3.30. A numerical example illustrating double transformation of binary variables into continue data from successive CA and standardized PCA applications. The three principle components (PCs) P_1-P_3 of PCA will be used as regression variables to develop a predictive model of concentrations. The most influent binary variables to PCs will be identified by a sensitivity analysis.

At this stage, the question of continue data was solved, but the new continue predictive data and the concentration variable (to predict) are associated to two different metric spaces, viz. Chi-2 and Euclidean, respectively. Therefore, it becomes required to bring back the predictive data to a same metric space than the predicted ones (the concentrations): for that, CA factorial coordinates F_{ij} will be brought back to Euclidean space by applying a standardized PCA (Figure 3.30c). The factorial coordinate F_{ij} of each individual i along the direction of each eigenvector U_j (j=1 to p-1) will be standardized with respect to the mean $\overline{F}_j$ and standard deviation Sd_{Fj} of the corresponding factor F_j (Eq. 3.16):

$$ y_{ij} = \frac{F_{ij} - \overline{F}_j}{Sd_{F_j}} \qquad (3.16) $$

In addition to the transfer of patterns from χ^2 to Euclidean space, such a transformation has the advantage to standardize the different factors F_j to unit variances. This avoids that the highest variability factors (the first ones F_1, F_2, ...) hide the lowest variability factors (the last ones ..., F_{p-1}).

Standardized PCA applied on the factorial coordinates of CA gives p-1 new columns of factorial coordinates called principle components (PCs) ($P_1...P_{p-1}$) and varying in Euclidean space (Figure 3.30c). Such PCs can be used as appropriate variables to build regression model predicting the concentrations of a given metabolite (Figures 3.30d, 3.31a).

II.8.2.5. Principle Component-Based Regression Modeling

Concentrations of a given metabolite can be predicted by a regression model based on the different PCs (P_k) as well as their interactions (Antoniewicz et al., 2006). For that different models exist, viz.:

- Full factorial model: f(A, B, C, AB, AC, BC, ABC)
- interaction model: f(A, B, C, AB, AC, BC)
- Square model: f(A, B, C, A², B², C²)

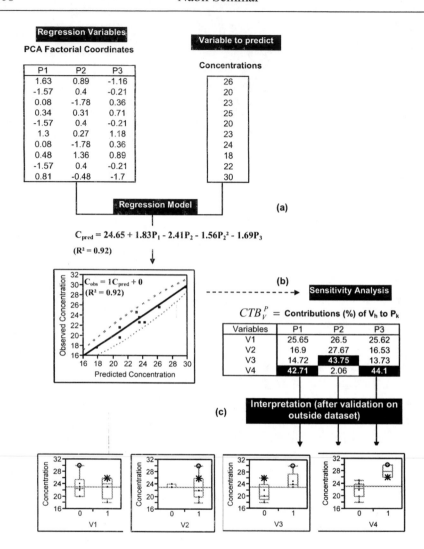

Figure 3.31. Development and interpretation of regression model predicting concentrations from principle components P_1-P_3 issued from a double transformation of initial binary variables by successive CA-PCA applications.

Eventually, a better multi-linear regression model could be obtained by an appropriate data transformation (e.g. log, inverse, square root, etc.) rather than the crude values. In summary, different regression models need to be compared, then the best one can be judged on the basis of two criteria: a final model can be selected on the basis of (i) a minimal number of significant regression variables giving (ii) a high determination coefficient R^2 (e.g. $R^2 \geq$

0.6). For that, a backward stepwise regression can be applied by introducing all the explanative variables (PCs) and their interactions, then by eliminating step by step those having negligible effect on the R^2 value. Thus, a few number of significant regression variables (PCs, interactions and/or squares) can be retained to predict correctly the concentration of the considered metabolite. In the numerical example of figure 3.30, a square model was applied to predict concentration in relation to P_1, P_2, P_3, P_1^2, P_2^2, P_3^2. After elimination of the not significant variables P_1^2 and P_3^2, the resulting model was: C= 24.65 + 1.83P_1 − 2.41P_2 − 1.56P_2^2 - 1.69P_3 with a determination coefficient R^2=0.92 (Figure 3.31a).

Finally, such a model needs to be validated on external data to be considered as reliable or useful to other experimental datasets. In such a validation case and only in such a case, the model results will be interpreted.

II.8.2.6. Validation of Regression Model

The regression model predicts concentrations from PCs (P_k) given by a PCA applied on the CA factorial coordinates of initial binary data. The validation of such CA-PCA-regression model requires its application on external or foreign dataset which did not contribute to the model building:

External binary data are subjected to the previous CA model to calculate their factorial coordinates. The resulting CA coordinates will be given to the previous PCA model to calculate their corresponding PCA coordinates. Finally, the calculated PCs will be used in the already built regression model to calculate the predicted concentration values. The regression model will be validated if the scatter plot of observed vs predicted concentrations has a well stretched shape with acceptable determination coefficient (e.g. R^2>0.45).

II.8.2.7. Interpretation of PCs-Based Regression Model

The predictive regression model will be interpreted in terms of effects of the initial binary variables (e.g. genetic variables) on metabolite concentrations. For that, a sensitivity analysis is needed to determine what binary variables are the most contributive to the significant PCs in the regression model (Figures 3.31b; 3.30e):

By applying a standardized PCA on the factors F_j of CA, one obtains new factorial coordinates defining the PCs P_k: along each P_k, each factor F_j will have a coordinate $P_k(F_j)$. To determine what F_j is/are the most influent on a given P_k, one calculates the contribution of each F_j to P_k:

$$C_{F_j}^{P_k} = \frac{P_k^2(F_j)}{\lambda_k} \tag{3.17}$$

Where:

$P_k^2(F_j)$: the square of factorial coordinate of factor F_j along the PC P_k.

λ_k : the eigenvalue of PC P_k.

$C_{F_j}^{P_k}$: the contribution of factor variable F_j to the PC P_k. Formula (3.17) is applied to PCA results.

A higher absolute value of $C_{F_j}^{P_k}$ indicates a more influent factor F_j to principle component P_k.

Similarly to the PCs P_k, the CA factors (F_j) are latent variables combining all the initial binary variables V_h. By the same way than Eq. 3.17, the contribution $C_{V_h}^{F_j}$ of each binary variable to each factor F_j can be calculated by:

$$C_{V_h}^{F_j} = \frac{V_{+h}}{V_{++}} \cdot \frac{F_j^2(V_h)}{\lambda_j} \tag{3.18}$$

Where:

$F_j^2(V_h)$: Square of factorial coordinate of binary variable V_h along the factor F_j.

λ_j : Eigenvalue of factor F_j.

V_{+h}: Sum of all the values of column h of disjonctive table D.

V_{++}: Sum of all the values of table D.

The ratio V_{+h}/V_{++} represents the mass or weight of column V_h in table D. However, in standardized PCA, the formula (Eq. 3.17) is simplified because one attributes a unit mass (=1) to each column (F_j).

Absolute contribution of binary variable V_h to factor F_j given by CA. Formula (3.18) is applied on CA results.

Higher is the absolute value of $C_{V_h}^{F_j}$, more important is the contribution of initial variable V_h to factor F_j.

By the fact that PCs are not directly linked to the binary variables V_h, the contribution of V_h to P_k can be determined by means of a sensitivity analysis that can be generally expressed by a differential equation:

$$\frac{dP_k}{dV_h} = \frac{dP_k}{dF_j} \cdot \frac{dF_j}{dV_h} \qquad\qquad (3.19)$$

Such contributions can be calculated by means of the product between the contribution matrix ($CTB_{V_h}^{F_j}$) of V_h to F_j in CA and the contribution matrix ($CTB_{F_j}^{P_k}$) of F_j to P_k in PCA (Figures 3.30e, 3.31b):

$$(CTB_{V_h}^{P_k}) = (CTB_{V_h}^{F_j}) \times (CTB_{F_j}^{P_k}) \qquad\qquad (3.20)$$

The resulting matrix $CTB_{V_h}^{P_k}$ gives the contribution levels of each initial binary variable V_h (e.g. genetic variable) to the different PCs P_k. Therefore, the interpretation of each latent variable P_k can be carried out taking into account its most contributive variable(s) V_h. In the numerical example of figure 3.31, binary variables V_3 and V_4 appear as the most contributive to the three PCs P_1-P_3: Variable V_3 contributes to 43% of the construction of P_2, whereas V_4 contributes to 42.71 and 44.10% to P_1 and P_3, respectively (Figure 3.31b).

From contributions calculated by sensitivity analysis, the predictive model of concentrations from PCs can be interpreted in terms of the question: "how do the qualitative characaters V_h (eg. different genes) influence the concentrations of considered metabolite?" By reference to figure 3.31, the concentration variability seems to be mainly controlled by variables V_3 and V_4 where modalities 1 and 0 show increasing and decreasing effects on concentrations, respectively (box plots) (Figure 3.31c). Such observations can suggest that predictions in concentrations are influenced by a clustering effects of V_3 and V_4 generating two different variation ranges of concentrations. However, variables V_1 and V_2 which seem to have merging effects on concentrations showed lesser influences on the predictions.

Finally, the fact that PCs are latent variables (combining several initial variables), their signs in the regression model can't be attributed to a single initial variable leading to a non-interpretability.

Chapter 4

DISTANCES - AND SIMILARITY INDICES-BASED APPROACHES: CLUSTER ANALYSIS

I. AIM AND GENERAL METHODOLOGICAL CONCEPTS

Cluster analysis (ClA), also called data segmentation aims at partition of set of experimental units (e.g. set of metabolic profiles) into two or more homogeneous subsets called clusters. More precisely, it is a classification method for grouping individuals or objects into well distinct clusters so that the objects in the same cluster are more similar to one another than to objects in other clusters. In summary, internal cohesion and external distinction of clusters represent the fundamental criteria in ClA. Moreover, the concept of hierarchy between clusters can be considered by appropriate methods.

The resulting clusters can provide information on different trends which can have functional or evolutive meaning within the studied population. Thus, ClA represents a powerful tool to population analysis by structuring highly variable individual profiles (behaviors) in a population into a few number of homogeneous and interpretable clusters (trends) (Maharjan and Ferenci, 2005; Semmar et al., 2005; Everitt et al., 2001; Gordon, 1999; Dimitriadou et al., 2004; Jain et al., 1999; Milligan and Cooper, 1987).

The general methodology of ClA can be summarized by two iterative steps: (a) computation of distances between all the individual pairs to quantify the closeness/remoteness degrees between individual cases; (b) grouping the most similar (the less distant) cases into homogeneous subsets (clusters) according to a certain criterion (Figure 4.1). Different classification typologies can be obtained by using different distance kinds combined with different aggregation criteria. This provides several clustering structures which can be validated on the basis of their interpretation in biological (metabolic) terms.

There are many clustering techniques which can be classified under two general approaches: hierarchical and non-hierarchical approaches:

Hierarchical methods provide hierarchical partitions in which the members of inferior-ranking clusters become members of larger, higher-ranking clusters. Intuitively, such structures are analogous to that of leaves-branches-trunk in a tree (Figure 4.2a). They are obtained by optimizing the hierarchical attachment ways between elements and higher-rank classes (Legendre and Legendre, 2000). Consequently, they have the advantage to provide classifications which highlight relationships between clusters.

Non-hierarchical methods provide a single partition of n individuals into q groups by optimizing the within-group homogeneity. Intuitively, the single partition structure is analogous to that of different geographical areas separated by frontiers (Figure 4.2b). Non-hierarchical classification can be applied when the aim is to obtain a global representation of direct associations between the elements instead of a summary of their hierarchies. Thus, they provide more simple representations than hierarchical methods. Also, they are less computation expensive than hierarchical methods, and consequently their application is particularly more appropriate on very large datasets (e.g. 5000 individuals). However, by opposition to the hierarchical methods, they provide limited information on the relative states of individuals, and on the relationships between clusters.

In metabolomics, CIA helps to analyse complex variability of metabolomic dataset. This is all the more important since the metabolic profiles in a dataset can vary gradually by slight fluctuations in the relative levels of their metabolites, resulting in the absence of frank borders between profiles. Apart from the statistical delimitation of groups within studied population, CIA explores the continuum in variability of metabolic profiles to extract relevant information on their hierarchical organization and relative differentiation degrees.

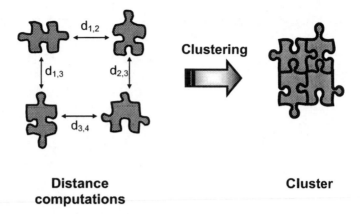

**Distance
computations**

Cluster

Figure 4.1. Intuitive presentation of the two main steps in cluster analysis: distance computations and clustering.

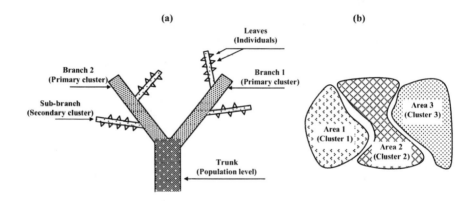

Figure 4.2. Intuitive presentation of two clustering approaches. (a) hierarchical clustering; (b) non-hierarchical or partitional clustering.

II. HIERARCHICAL CLUSTER ANALYSIS

II.1. Background on General Techniques

Hierarchical cluster analysis (HCA) includes several clustering techniques which can be subdivided into divisive (top-down) and agglomerative (bottom-up) methods (Figure 4.3) (Lance and Williams, 1967):

Divisive method, less common, starts with a single cluster containing all the objects. Then, it successively splits clusters until only clusters of individual objects remain. Although some divisive techniques attempt to minimize the within-cluster square error sum, they face problems of computational complexity that are not easy to overcome (Milligan and Cooper, 1987).

Agglomerative method starts with every single object in a single cluster. Then, in a series of successive iterations, it agglomerates (merges) the closest pair of clusters by satisfying some similarity criterion, until all of the data is in one cluster. The agglomerative method is the one especially described in this chapter.

The complete process of agglomerative hierarchical clustering requires defining an inter-individual distance and an inter-cluster linkage criterion. These two points represent the basis of a two-steps iterative process:

1. Calculation of the (dis)similarities or distances between all individual cases;
2. Fusion of the most appropriate (close, similar) clusters by using a clustering algorithm, and then recalculate the distances.

These two steps are repeated until all cases are in one cluster.

Finally, the hierarchical classification given by HCA is graphically represented by a tree of clusters, called dendrogram (Figure 4.3).

II.2. Dissimilarity Measures

Dissimilarities are calculated to quantify separation degrees between points. On continuous data, distances are calculated to evaluate dissimilarities between individuals. However, on qualitative data (binary, counts), the dissimilarities are indirectly evaluated from similarity indices (SI) which can be transformed into dissimilarities by single operations, e.g. (1–SI). A part from distances and SI, there are many ways to measure a dissimilarity/similarity according to circumstances and data type: correlation coefficient, non metric coefficient, cosine, information-gain or entropy-loss (Everitt, et al., 2001; Gordon, 1999; Arabie et al., 1996; Lance and Williams, 1967; Shannon, 1948).

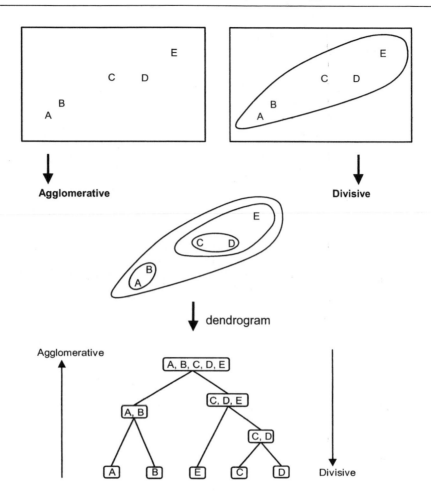

Figure 4.3. Two tree-building protocols in hierarchical cluster analysis (HCA) consisting in grouping (agglomerative method) or separating (divisive method) progressively individuals.

II.2.1. Continuous Data and Distance Computations

II.2.1.1. Euclidean Distance

Euclidean distance is appropriately used to calculate remoteness between profiles containing continuous data. It is a particular case of Minkowski metric:

$$dist(x_i, x_k) = \left[\sum_{j=1}^{p} \left| x_{ij} - x_{kj} \right|^r \right]^{1/r}$$ (4.1)

where:

- r is an exponent parameter defining a distance type (=1 for Manhattan distance, =2 for Euclidean distance, etc.);
- x_{ij}, x_{kj} are values of variable j for the objects i and i' respectively;
- p is the total number of variables describing the profiles x_i, x_k.
- j, i, i': indices of variables (j=1 to p) and profiles i and i', respectively.

Let's give a numerical example of three concentration profiles containing three metabolites:

	Metabolites		
Profiles	M1	M2	M3
X1	10	6	4
X2	10	4	3
X3	5	3	2

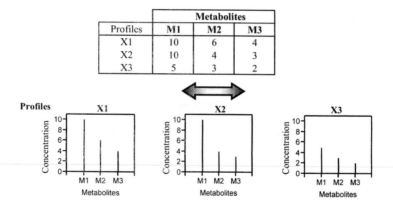

By applying the Euclidean distance, one would know what are the two closest profiles? To respond to this question, we have to calculate three distances between pairs of profiles: X_1-X_2, X_1-X_3 and X_2-X_3:

	Metabolites j				Euclidean distances d
Profiles i, i' $(X_i - X_{i'})^2$	M1	M2	M3	Sum	d=√Sum= $\sqrt{\sum_{j=1}^{p=3}(X_{ij}-X_{i'j})^2}$
$(X_1$-$X_2)^2$	0	4	1	5	2.24
$(X_1$-$X_3)^2$	25	9	4	38	6.16
$(X_2$-$X_3)^2$	25	1	1	27	5.20

From the lowest Euclidean distance, one can deduce that profiles X_1 and X_2 are the closest between them, whereas X_1 and X_3 are the farthest.

The distance can be calculated either on crude data or after data transformation. Calculation on crude data is appropriate when the variables have comparable variances or when one would attribute domination to higher variance variable. In the other case, data transformation can be used to attribute comparable scales and equal influences to the variables in cluster analysis. The most common transformation (standardization) consists of the conversion of crude data into standard scores (z-scores) by subtracting the mean and dividing by the standard deviation of each variable.

Many other distance measures are appropriate according to the data types: Mahalanobis, Hellinger, Chi-square distance, etc. (Blackwood et al., 2003; Gibbons and Roth, 2002).

II.2.1.2. Chi-Square Distance

Chi-square (χ^2) distance is applied on dataset the values of which are additive both on rows and columns. This is the case for concentration datasets which are common in metabolomics. This distance can be calculated according to the formula:

$$\chi^2(X_1, X_2) = \sum_{j=1}^{p} \frac{Sum_{tot}}{Sum_j} \left(\frac{X_{1j}}{Sum_{X_1}} - \frac{X_{2j}}{Sum_{X_2}} \right)^2 \tag{4.2}$$

where :

X_1, X_2 denotes individual profiles (e.g. metabolic profile).

j: index of variable j (e.g. metabolite j).

X_{1j}, X_{2j}: values of variables j in the profiles X_1 and X_2, respectively.

Sum_{X1}, Sum_{X2} are the sums of values of all the variables in each individual X_1 and X_2, respectively.

Sum_j is the sum of the values of variable j in all the profiles of dataset (e.g. sum of concentrations of metabolite j).

Sum_{tot} is the sum of all the values of the whole dataset.

According to the χ^2 distance, two individuals are all the more close since their relative profiles are similar. This similarity based on relative values can be checked when the respective values of two profiles are multiple the ones of others.

Let's calculate the χ^2 distances between the three profiles X_1, X_2, X_3 (Figure 4.4). The computations show that the minimal χ^2 distance concerns the pairs (X_1, X_3) by opposition to the Euclidean distance. This χ^2 is minimal, indeed null, because the absolute profiles X_1 (10, 6, 4) and X_3 (5, 3, 2) correspond to the same relative profile (0.5, 0.3, 0.2).

II.2.2. Qualitative Variables and Similarity Indices

For qualitative data (binary, counting), many similarity indices (SI) can be used as intuitive measures of the closeness between individuals: Jaccard, Sorensen-Dice, Tanimoto, Sokal-Michener indices, etc. (Jaccard , 1912; Duatre et al., 1999; Rouvray, 1992). The similarity indices are less sensitive to the null values of the variables, and thus they are useful in the case of sparse data. To evaluate similarity between two individuals X_1 and X_2, we need three or four essential elements (a-c, d): a = number of shared characteristics; b = number of characteristics present in X_1 and absent in X_2; c = number of characteristics present in X_2 and absent in X_1; d = number of characteristics absent both in X_1 and X_2 (required for some SI).

The different *SI* can be converted into dissimilarity *D* according to the formula:

$$D = 1 - SI \quad \text{if SI} \in [0, 1] \tag{4.3}$$

$$D = \frac{1 - SI}{2} \quad \text{if SI} \in [-1, 1] \tag{4.4}$$

To illustrate the concept of similarity index, let's give a numerical example concerning three metabolic profiles characterized by 10 metabolites the concentration of which are not known (Figure 4.5). In such case, quantitative data (concentrations) are not available, and consequently, distances can't be computed. Experimentally, metabolite spot profiles can be routinely obtained by appropriate analytical techniques such as thin layer chromatography or electrophoresis. Therefore, information on presence/absence of metabolites j in the different profiles X_i can be used to calculate SI between the profiles. Calculations are showed for the pair of profiles (X_1, X_2) (Figure 4.5).

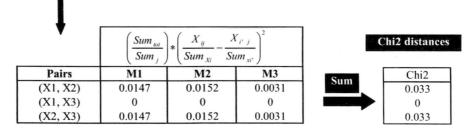

Figure 4.4. Numerical example illustrating the computation of Chi2 distances between three pairs of profiles.

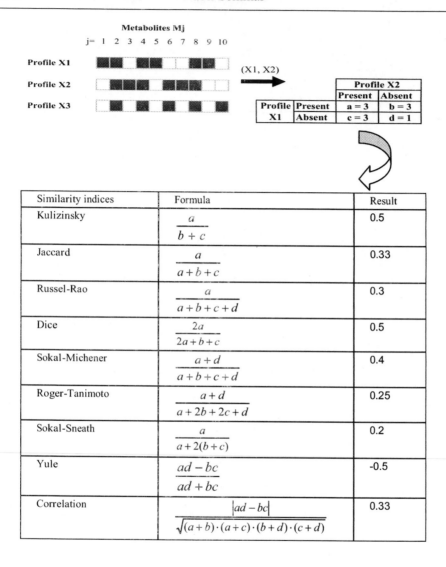

Figure 4.5. Calculus of similarity between two profiles according to different similarity indices.

II.3. Clustering Techniques

After computation of distances or dissimilarities between all the individuals of the dataset (e.g. metabolic profiles), it becomes possible to merge them into homogeneous and well separated groups by using an aggregation rule: initially, the most close (the less distant) individuals are merged to give a cluster. After the apparition of some small clusters, the immediate next step consists in merging the most similar clusters into larger clusters by reference to a certain homogeneity criterion (aggregation rule). Such procedure is iteratively applied until all the individuals/clusters are merged into one entity; the most separated (most dissimilar) clusters will be merged at the final step of the clustering procedure. This leads to a hierarchical stratification of the whole population into well homogeneous and separated clusters.

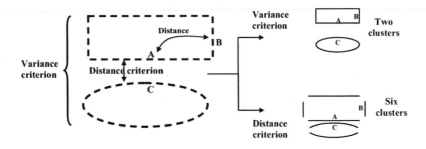

Figure 4.6. Intuitive representation of clustering based on distance and on variance criteria.

Clustering techniques include several aggregation rules which are based on different homogeneity criteria. Two clustering principles will be illustrated here: distance-based (a) and variance-based (b) clustering (Figure 4.6). The distance-based clustering will be illustrated by four aggregation rules: single, average, centroid and complete links (Figure 4.7); the variance-based clustering will be illustrated by the second order moment rule (or Ward algorithm) (Figure 4.8) (Ward, 1963; Everitt, 2001; Gordon, 1999; Arabie, 1996).

Using the distance criterion, let's consider:

- r and s, two clusters with n_r and n_s elements respectively,
- x_{ri} and x_{sk}, the ith and k^{th} elements in clusters r and s, respectively,
- $D(r, s)$, the inter-cluster distance.

It is assumed that $D(r, s)$ is the smallest calculated distance in the system, so that r and s fuse to form a new cluster t with n_t ($=n_r+n_s$) elements:

II.3.1. Single Link Rule

In single-link, two clusters (r and s) are merged if they have the two closest objects (nearest neighbors) (Figure 4.7). In this case, the minimal distance $D(r, s)$ is between the closest individuals of clusters r and s.

Single-link rule strings objects together to form clusters, and consequently it tends to give elongated chain clusters. This elongation is due to the tendency to incorporate intermediate objects into an existing cluster rather than to form a new one. A single linkage algorithm would perform well when clusters are naturally elongated.

II.3.2. Complete Link Rule

In complete-link, two clusters are merged if their farthest objects are separated by a minimal distance compared with all the distances between the farthest neighbors of all the clusters (Figure 4.7). This rule leads to minimize the distance between the most distant objects in the new cluster.

Complete-link rule results in dilatation and may produce many clusters. This algorithm is known to give well compact clusters and usually performs well when the objects form naturally distinct "clumps", or when one wishes to emphasize discontinuities (Jain et al., 1999; Milligan and Cooper, 1987). Moreover, if unequal size clusters are present in the data, complete-link gives superior recovery than other algorithms (Milligan and Cooper, 1987). Complete-link, however, suffers from the opposite defect of single-link: it tends "to break" groups presenting a certain lengthening in space, so as to provide rather spherical (rather than elongated) classes.

II.3.3. Centroid Link Rule

In centroid-link, a cluster is represented by its mean position (i.e. centroid). The joining between clusters will be based on the smallest distance between their centroids (Figure 4.7). This method is a compromise between single and complete linkages.

The centroid method is more robust to outliers than other hierarchical methods, but in other respects, this method can produce a cluster tree that is not monotonic. This occurs when the distance from the union of two clusters, r and s, to a third cluster u is less than the distance from either r or s to u. In this case, sections of the dendrogram change direction. This change is an indication that one should use another clustering rule.

II.3.4. Average Link Rule

In average-link rule, the closest clusters are those having the minimal average distance calculated between all their point pairs. The basic assumption regarding this rule is that all the elements in a cluster contribute to the inter-cluster similarity.

Average linkage is also an interesting compromise between the nearest and the farthest neighbors methods. Average linkage tends to join clusters with small variances; it is slightly biased toward producing clusters with "equal" variances. The agglomeration levels can be difficult to interpret with this method.

II.3.5. Variance Criterion Based Clustering: Ward Method

Ward's method (also called incremental sum of squares method) is distinct from all the other clustering methods because it uses an analysis of variance to evaluate the distances between centroids of clusters; it builds clusters by optimizing the ratio of between- on within-cluster variances (Figure 4.8).

Initially, the set of n separated points represents a situation where the variances between- and within-classes are maximal and minimal, respectively, because each element is considered as one class, viz. n distinct classes of null variance in all (Figure 4.8a). When the points are progressively merged into clusters, the variance within-class (or intra-class variance) increases at the expense of the variance between classes (or inter-class variance). To optimize clustering under such unfavorable and unavoidable fact, Ward's algorithm selects at each step, the clustering under which the lost of inter-class variance is minimal. In other words, at a given clustering step, two (children) clusters are merged if they result in the smallest increase in variance within the new single (mother) cluster (Duatre et al., 1999) (Figure 4.8). After comparison of all the pairs of clusters intended to aggregation, Ward's rule merges the pair (r, s) with the minimum value of $D(r, s)$ representing the lost part of inter-class variance:

$$D(r,s) = \frac{d^2\left(\overline{x_r}, \overline{x_s}\right)}{\left(\dfrac{1}{n_r} + \dfrac{1}{n_s}\right)} = \frac{1}{\left(\dfrac{1}{n_r} + \dfrac{1}{n_s}\right)} (\overline{x_r} - \overline{x_s})' \; (\overline{x_r} - \overline{x_s}) \qquad (4.5)$$

where:

n_r, n_s : total numbers of objects (weights) of clusters r and s, respectively ;

$D(r, s)$: part of inter-class variance lost if clusters r and s are merged;

$\overline{x}_r$, $\overline{x}_s$: coordinates of the centroids of clusters r and s respectively;

$d(\overline{x}_r, \overline{x}_s)$: distance between the centroids of clusters r and s .

Ward's method is regarded as very efficient and gives clearly interpretable agglomeration levels. However, it tends to give balanced clusters of small size, and it is sensitive to outliers (Milligan, 1980).

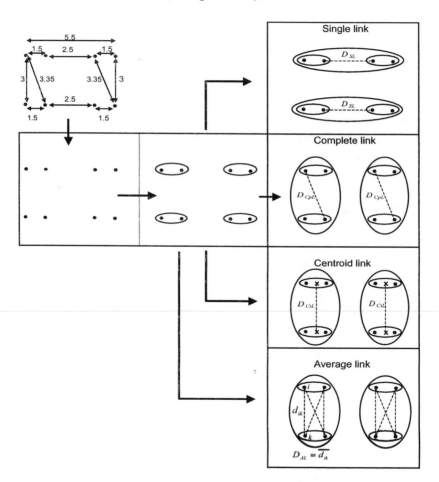

Figure 4.7. Schematic representations of different clustering rules in agglomerative cluster analysis. D_{SL}, D_{CpL}, D_{CtL}, D_{AL}: Minimal distances used in single, complete, centroid and average link, respectively. d_{ik}: distance between elements i and k belonging to two different clusters. $\overline{d}_{ik}$: average distance calculated on all the distances between all the pairs of points i and k.

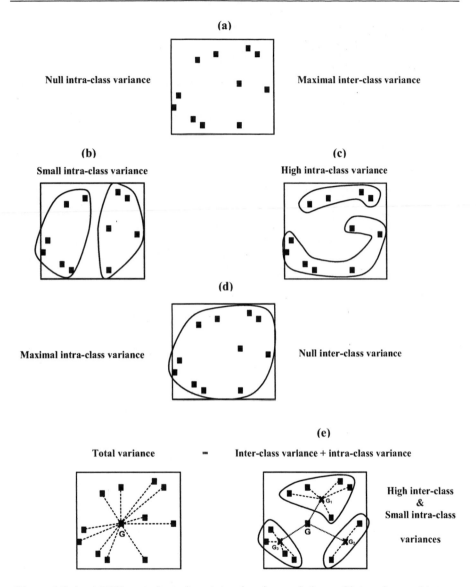

Figure 4.8. (a-e) Different clustering states showing variations of intra-class and inter-class variances the one at the expense of the other. (e) Clustering corresponding to a high ratio (inter-/intra-class variances), given by Ward's algorithm by minimizing the lost of inter-class variance at all the successive aggregation steps. Legend: G: centroid or gravity centre of the whole dataset; G1, G2, G3: centroids of clusters 1, 2, 3, respectively.

II.4. Identification and Interpretation
of Clusters from Dendrogram

After clustering of all the individuals according to a given criterion, HCA provides a dendrogram which is a tree-like diagram informing about the classification structure of the population (Figure 4.9). In the dendrogram, a certain number of clusters can be retained on the basis of high homogeneity and separation levels. For each cluster, the homogeneity and separation levels of each cluster can be graphically evaluated on the dendrogram from its compactness and distinctness, respectively:

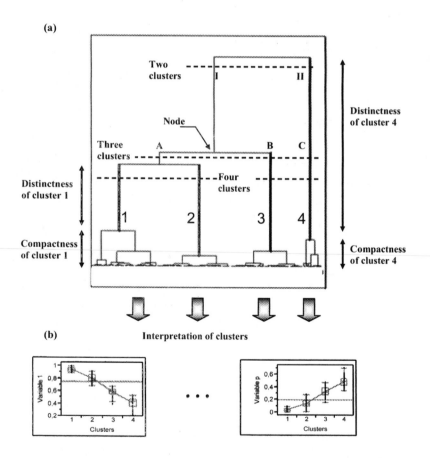

Figure 4.9. Illustration of the different parameters required for the identification and interpretation of clusters in a dendrogram.

In a dendrogram (Figure 4.9a), the number of clusters increases from the top to the bottom. This number is often empirically determined by how many vertical lines are cut by a horizontal line. Raising or lowering the horizontal line decreases or increases the number of cut vertical lines, respectively, i.e. the number clusters resulting from the subdivision of the population. Validation of resulting clusters depends on whether they have a clear biological (e.g. clinical) meaning or not.

The dissimilarity level or distance between two clusters or two subunits is determined from the height of the node that joins them. This height represents also the compactness of the parent cluster formed by merging the two children clusters. In other words, the compactness of a cluster represents the minimum distance at which the cluster comes into existence (Figure 4.9a). At the lowest levels of dendrogram, the subunits are individuals.

When the classification is well structured, each cluster contains individuals which are similar between them and dissimilar with regard to the individuals of other clusters. It results in clusters with low compactness and long distinct branches (high distinctness). The distinctness of a cluster is the distance from the point (node) at which it comes into existence to the point at which it is merged into a larger cluster.

The interpretation of distinct clusters can be easily guided by box-plots highlighting the dispersions of the p initial variables (e.g. the p metabolites) in the different identified clusters (Figure 4.9b). These graphics help to detect which variable(s) significantly influences the distinction between clusters. This step serves to determine the meaning of each cluster.

III. NON-HIERARCHICAL CLUSTERING METHODS

III.1. Background on General Techniques

Non-hierarchical clustering (NHC) or partitional methods consist in finding a single partition of a set of objects into q groups or clusters such that the elements within each cluster are similar to one another than to objects in the other cluster (Figure 4.2b) (Jain and Dubes, 1988).

There are several NHC methods based on different principles and criteria among which one can cite square error- and graph theoretic-based methods. Square error partition will be illustrated here by the K-means method which can be considered as the simplest NHC (McQueen, 1967).

III.2. K-Means Clustering Method

The K-means clustering method is based on the iteration of two successive steps consisting in (1) partitioning the n points into K initial sets followed by (2) the calculation of the mean point (centroid) of each set. At each iteration of step (1), the algorithm calculates new partitions by associating each input point to the closest centroid by using Euclidean distance. In step (2), the centroids of clusters are recalculated taking into account the new partitions given by step (1). The iteration of steps (1) and (2) continue until convergence, i.e. until there is no assignment of any individual from one cluster to another, or until the squared error ceases to decrease significantly after some number of iterations.

Such a methodology will be detailed in the next sections and illustrated in Figure 4.10:

1. The K-means algorithm requires initially the specification of the number K of clusters that will be established by NHC to classify the n individuals of the population. In the example of figure 4.10, the number K was initially fixed to 2 clusters in which $n=8$ individuals will be partitioned (Figures 4.10a, b). The number K can be defined on the basis of fundamental biological knowledges or from the number of trends highlighted by a previous multivariate ordination analysis (e.g. PCA or CA).
2. To start, each cluster j ($j=1$ to K) will be initially located by arbitrary coordinates of its centroid G_j (Figure 4.10b). The K centroids can be chosen visually, randomly or heuristically: for example, they can correspond to centroids of K clusters previously given by a HCA. The K points G_j are called mobile centres because their positions will change in the next steps under the effect of the masses of points contained in the temporary clusters.
3. From the K initial arbitrary centroids, K distances are calculated between each of the n points and these K centroids G_j. Then, the minimal distance among the K ones will affect the points to appropriate initial cluster j (Figure 4.10c). The K obtained clusters satisfy a minimal sum of squared errors e^2 between all the points x_i and their respective centroids G_j (Eq. 4.6):

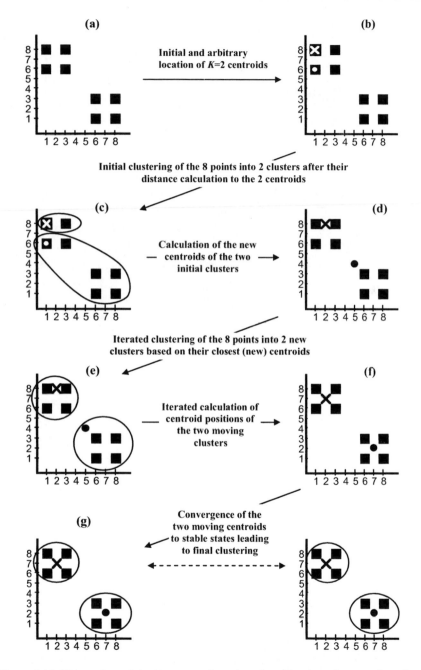

Figure 4.10. Illustration of the K-means clustering algorithm based on two iterative processes consisting in calculating moving centroids and delimitations of their corresponding clusters.

$$e_l^2 = \sum_{j=1}^{K} \sum_{i=1}^{n_j} (x_i^{(j)} - G_j)^2$$

(4.6)

Where $x_i^{(j)}$ is the ith element belonging to the jth cluster and G_j is the centroid of the jth cluster; the index l corresponds to the numerous of the considered iteration (Jain, 1999). After the first iterations of NHC (Figure 4.10c), the minimization of e_l^2 gives generally a local and not global (or absolute) minimum. Next iterations lead to reach the global minimum which corresponds to the final (stable) clustering state. Such a minimization criterion corresponds to the objective function "within-group variance" which is the same as in Ward's agglomerative clustering method (Chapter 4, II.3.5). However, in K-means algorithm such a minimization is more direct because NHC methods optimize directly the within-group homogeneity, whereas the Ward's method optimizes the hierarchical attachment ways between elements leading indirectly to a minimal within-group variance. Moreover, the number of group is not specified *a priori* in Ward's algorithm.

4. The K delimited groups define new centroids G_j which will be calculated (Figure 4.10d). The change in positions of centroids G_j is due to the variation of masses of points of clusters at successive iterations. These variations will be progressively attenuated leading to stabilize the centroid positions (Figures 4.10e-g).
5. The distance between each input point and each centroid (G_l to G_k) will be calculated, then the point i will be affected to the closest centroid (as step 3). The resulting partitions obtained successively (step 5 following step 3) vary markedly at the first iterations, then they will be progressively stabilize under the effect of the masses of neighbour points (convergence) (Figure 4.10e).
6. The centroids G_j of the new clusters are calculated (iterated step 4) (Figure 4.10f), and the process will be iterated until the within-group homogeneity (variance) will stabilize, i.e. the centroid positions becomes unchanged (Figure 4.10g).
   After convergence, the within-group variance (e^2) (Eq. 4.6) reaches a minimal value, but it is needed to check that such a value doesn't correspond to a local minimum (instead of the searched global

minimum) (Figure 4.11). This checking is a general rule to apply in optimization problems to avoid that arbitrary initial conditions influence the final results. For that, it is advised to repeat several times the K-means algorithm by starting from new arbitrary initial partitions (different initial centroid locations): if the process give the same result, the final partition can be considered as acceptable, i.e. corresponding to the global minimum of squared error e^2 (Figure 4.11). If different final results are obtained from different initial partitions, one retains the result corresponding to the minimal intra-class variance.

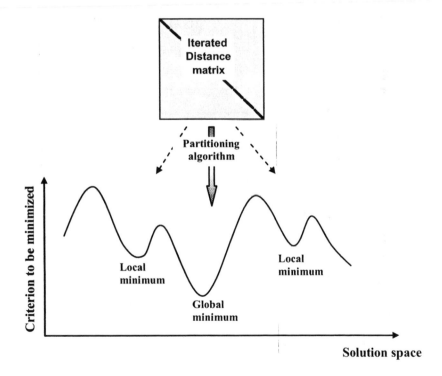

Figure 4.11: Graphical representation of objective function to be minimized by searching its global minimum and by avoiding local minima. In K-mean algorithm, the distance matrix contains the distances of the n input points to the K centroids obtained at each iteration step. Apart from the distances, different minimization algorithms can use other objective functions to minimize (e.g. inverse of probability, i.e. probability maximization).

III.3. K-Means method: Advantages and Limits

K-means method is popular by its simplicity and rapidity requiring just one parameter to be set (the number of clusters). It has the advantage to optimize a single dispersion criterion consisting of the second order moment of a partition. However, the final clustering result is not guaranteed to correspond to the absolute optimum (i.e. the best solution). This requires the application of the K-means algorithm several times with different initial partitions. This method can be helpfully used in conjunction with other clustering methods (Pierens et al., 2005).

Chapter 5

OUTLIERS AND EXTREME CASES ANALYSIS

I. INTRODUCTION

Biological populations can be characterized by a high variability consisting of multiple dissimilarities between individuals. Beyond of such diversity, it is important to identify atypical individuals which can be considered as potential sources of heterogeneity. Detection of atypical individuals is useful to (Figure 5.1):

- Avoid working on heterogeneous dataset,
- Detect original/rare information which needs some particular consideration.

In summary, outliers can be either suspect values or represent interesting points which provide evidence of new phenomena or new populations. In all the cases, a dataset needs to be treated with and without its detected outliers; then comparisons will help to conclude on the diversity or heterogeneity of the studied population.

For example in metabolomics, some individuals can show atypical biosynthesis, secretion, storage or transformation (elimination) for certain metabolites compared to the whole population. In clinical middle, such cases need to be identified in order to optimize their treatments. Moreover in statistical analysis of biological populations, identification and removing of outliers allow to extract more reliable information on the variation space of studied population, because the presence of outliers in a dataset can be responsible for bias in the results: for instance, the mean of the population can be significantly shifted to higher values under the effect of some atypically high value(s). Also, a relationship between two variables (e.g. two metabolites) can be biased because of some miss-located points. Finally, extreme cases can represent original trends within population.

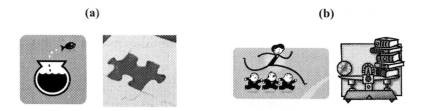

Figure 5.1. Intuitive examples illustrating two meaning of outliers; outliers can be suspect points resulting in biased results (a), or can provide original information on extreme states in the population or on new populations (b).

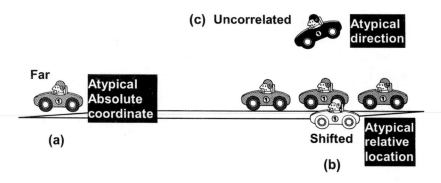

Figure 5.2. Intuitive representation of different types of outliers.

II. DIFFERENT TYPES OF OUTLIERS

Outliers can be defined according to three criteria: remoteness, gap, deflection (Figure 5.2).

- Remoteness concerns individuals (e.g. metabolic profiles) that are atypically far from the whole population because of atypically high or low coordinates (Figure 5.2a).
- Gap concerns individuals that are shifted within the population because of discordance in their coordinates (Figure 5.2b).
- Deflection concerns individuals that are not oriented along the global direction of the whole population (Figure 5.2c).

III. STATISTICAL CRITERIA TO IDENTIFICATION OF OUTLIERS

Identification of outliers is closely linked to the criterion under which the dissimilarities between individuals are evaluated. The greatest dissimilarities can help to detect the most atypical/original individuals. The three types of outliers presented in figure 5.2, can be identified from computations using three types of distances (Figure 5.3):

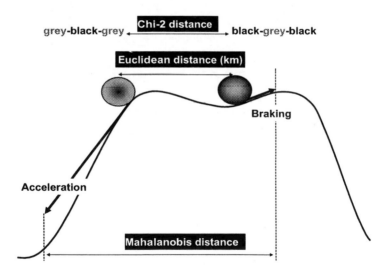

Figure 5.3. Illustration of three distance criteria to evaluate the outlier/non-outlier states of individuals within a population.

- Differences can be undertaken on the basis of measurable data (continue variables). Classic example is given by kilometric measurements leading to conclude about the remoteness of individuals to a reference point. Such remoteness is evaluated by means of Euclidean distance.

- Differences between individuals can be described on the basis of presence-absence for qualitative variables, or relative values for quantitative variables. In a given individual, the presences and absences of qualitative variables are compared to their respective total presences-absences in the population. Rarely present or absent characteristics in a given individual lead to consider such individual as atypical. The evaluation of atypical individuals on the basis of such relative states can be performed by means of the Chi-2 distance.

- Atypical individuals can be identified on the basis of their role to stretch, dilate and/or modify the global shape of a population. Stretching, dilatation levels and shape structure are statistically evaluated by means of variances and covariances. For that, the variance-covariance matrix of the whole population is considered as a metric to identify atypical individuals with atypical variation (shape) profiles. The distance calculated taking into account the variances-covariances corresponds to the Mahalanobis distance.

The three different criteria presented above show that the outlier concept is closely linked to the used distance.

IV. GRAPHICAL IDENTIFICATION
OF UNIVARIATE OUTLIERS

The simplest outlier identification method consists in analyzing the values of all the individuals for a given variable. In such case, the atypical individuals correspond only to range outliers because of their atypically high or low values of the considered variable (Figure 5.2a). Graphically, such outliers can be identified by means of box-plots as points located beyond the cut-off values defined by the whiskers' extremities (Figure 5.4) (Hawkins, 1980; Filzmoser et al., 2005). These two extremities are calculated by adding and subtracting (1.5 × inter-quartile range) to third and first quartiles, respectively.

V. GRAPHICAL IDENTIFICATION
OF BIVARIATE OUTLIERS

When two variables X, Y are considered, the dataset can be represented graphically by using a scatter plot Y versus X. In the case of linear model, three kinds of outliers can be detected on the scatter plot viz., range (a), spatial (b) and relationship (c) outliers (Rousseeuw and Leroy, 1987; Cerioli and Riani, 1999; Robinson, 2005) (Figure 5.5):

For (a), the high coordinates (x, y) of the point will inflate variances of both variables, but will have little effect on the correlation; in this case, the point (x, y) is a univariate outlier according to each variable X, Y, separately.

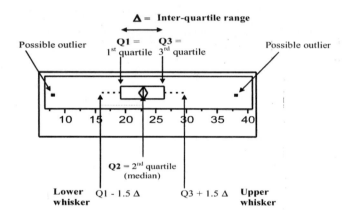

Figure 5.4. Tuckey Box-plot showing univariate outlier detection from the upper and/or lower limits of whiskers.

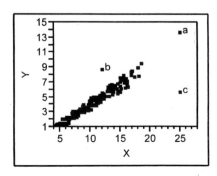

Figure 5.5. Graphical illustration of different types of outliers that can be detected from a scatter plot of two variables Y vs X.

Observation (b) is miss-located with respect to its neighboring values. It will have little effect on variances but will reduce the correlation.

For (c), outlier can be defined as an observation that falls outside of the expected area; it has a high moment (leverage point) through which it will reduce the correlation between Y and X, inflate the variance of X, but will have little effect on the variance of Y.

VI. IDENTIFICATION OF MULTIVARIATE OUTLIERS BASED ON DISTANCE COMPUTATIONS

When more than two variables are considered, the identification of outliers requires more computations on the multivariate matrix X (n rows × p columns) in which each element x_{ij} represents the value of variable j in individual i :

$$
X = \begin{pmatrix}
x_{11} & x_{12} & \cdots & x_{1j} & \cdots & x_{1p} \\
x_{21} & x_{22} & \cdots & x_{2j} & \cdots & x_{2p} \\
\cdots & \cdots & \cdots & \cdots & \cdots & \cdots \\
x_{i1} & x_{i2} & \cdots & x_{ij} & \cdots & x_{ip} \\
\cdots & \cdots & \cdots & \cdots & \cdots & \cdots \\
x_{n1} & x_{n2} & \cdots & x_{nj} & \cdots & x_{np}
\end{pmatrix} \quad i\,(1 \text{ to } n)
$$

$$j\,(1 \text{ to } p)$$

For that, appropriate metric distances have to be computed by combining all the variables X_j describing individuals i. In metabolomics, such a matrix can be represented by a dataset describing n metabolic profiles i by p metabolites j.

Distances are calculated by reference to a neutral profile representing a profound population state. Then, the calculated distances will be used to visualize the relative states of corresponding individuals within the population.

These distances are computed between individuals X_i and a reference individual X_0 by using three parameters: the coordinates x_{ij} and x_{0j} of the observed and reference individuals X_i and X_0, and a metric matrix Γ (Gnanadesikan and Kettenring, 1972; Barnett, 1976; Barnett and Lewis, 1994):

$$d^2(X_i, X_0) = \sum_{j=1}^{p}(x_{ij} - x_{0j})\Gamma^{-1}(x_{ij} - x_{0j})' \qquad (5.1)$$

The kind of distance depends on the matrix Γ:

- If Γ=identity matrix, d corresponds to the Euclidean distance;
- If Γ= matrix of the products (sum of lines × sum of columns), d corresponds to the Chi-2 distance;
- Γ=variance-covariance matrix, d corresponds to the Mahalanobis distance.

The use of these three distances allows identification of three kinds of outliers. For that, three graphical distance-based approaches can be used: Andrews curves (Andrews, 1972; Barnett, 1976; Everitt and Dunn, 1992), correspondence analysis (CA) (Greenacre, 1984, 1993; Mortier and Bar-Hen, 2004) and Jackknifed Mahalanobis distance (Swaroop and Winter, 1971; Robinson, 2005), respectively. These different methods provide complementary diagnostics on the states of individuals in a dataset, leading to extract different kinds outliers under different criteria: an outlier can be considered as much marked as it is identified by more diagnostics (Semmar et al., 2008).

Another approach used in multivariate data, consists in performing multiple regression analysis between a depend variable Y and several explanative ones X_j, then a scatter plot can be visualized between observed and predicted Y (Y_{obs} vs Y_{pred}) (Figure 5.5). However, this approach has the disadvantage to be model-dependent by opposition to the three distance-based approaches which advantageously extract independent-model outliers.

VI.1. Standard Mahalanobis Distance Computation

This section presents the basic concepts of the Mahalanobis distance (MD) computation; it will be followed by a presentation (§VI. 2) of the Jackknifed technique which is mainly used to calculate robust MD. The two techniques (ordinary and Jackknifed) will be illustrated by a numerical example.

The MD provides a multivariate measure of how much a profile is far from the centroid (average vector) of the whole database. Using Mahalanobis distance, we can assess how similar/dissimilar each profile x_i is to a profound (average) profile $\overline{x}$.

The MD takes into account the correlation structure of the data, and it is independent of the scales of the descriptive variables. It is computed as (Rousseeuw and Leroy, 1987):

$$MD_i^{\ 2} = (x_i - \overline{x})C^{-1}(x_i - \overline{x})'$$ (5.2)

Where:

$MD_i^{\ 2}$ is the squared Mahalanobis distance of the individual i from the average vector (or centroid) $\overline{x}(\overline{x_1}, \overline{x_2}, ..., \overline{x_j}, ..., \overline{x_p})$,

x_i: a p-row vector (x_{i1}, x_{i2}, ..., x_{ij}, ..., x_{ip}) representing individual i (e.g. patient i) characterized by p variables (e.g. p concentration values of a given metabolite measured at p time variables; or p concentrations of p metabolites measured at a given time).

$\overline{x}$: vector of the arithmetic means of the p variables

$$\overline{x} = \frac{1}{n}\sum_{i=1}^{n} x_i \text{ (with } n \text{ : total number of individuals)}$$ (5.3)

C: the covariance matrix of the p variables

$$C = \frac{1}{n-1}\sum_{i=1}^{n}(x_i - \overline{x})'(x_i - \overline{x})$$ (5.4)

The MD measures how far is each profile x_i from the average profile $\overline{x}$ in the variance-covariance metrics defined by C. Under Mahalanobis criterion, the remoteness from centroid $\overline{x}$ increases for profile x_i which increases variance(s) of variable(s) or decreases correlation(s) between them. Mahalanobis distance becomes Euclidean distance if the covariance matrix is replaced by the identity matrix. The purpose of these MD_i^2 is to detect observations for which the explanatory part lies far from that of the bulk of the data. By reference to formula 5.2, MD can increase by:

-   A great difference of x_{ij} to the mean $\overline{x}_j$ (high numerator).

- A weak variance s_j^2 of the variable j making the difference $(x_{ij} - \overline{x_j})$ to be more sensitive to the high values x_{ij}.
- Atypical variations $(x_{ij} - \overline{x_j})$ reducing correlation(s) between variable j and other variable(s); this results in decrease in covariance(s) (in denominator) and consequently increases MD.

Let's illustrate the MD calculation by a numerical example (Figure 5.6):

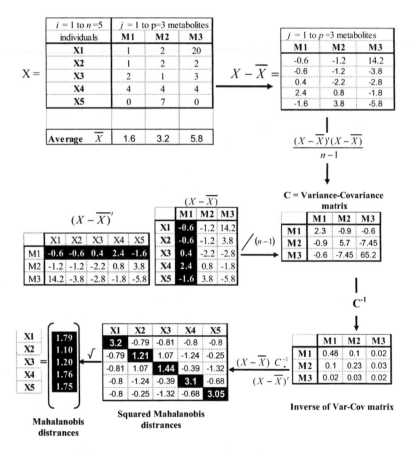

Figure 5.6. Numerical example illustrating the calculation of multivariate Mahalanobis distances.

The MD_i^2 values follow a chi-squared distribution with $(p-1)$ degrees of freedom (Hawkins, 1980). The multivariate outliers can be identified as points having Mahalanobis distances higher than the χ^2 cut-off value with a given alpha-risk (e.g. $\alpha \leq 0.05$) (Figure 5.7). Moreover, the most identical profiles to the centroid are those which have the lowest Mahalanobis distances; therefore, they can be considered as the most representative of the population (Figure 5.7; X_2, X_3 points). In our simple example, the number p of variables is equal to 3, and the freedom df is equal to $p-1=2$. For a α risk fixed to 5% ($\alpha=0.05$), the cut-off χ^2 value corresponding to df=2 is given by $\chi^2(2, 0.05)=5.99$. From the numerical example, no squared MD is higher than this cut-off value; consequently, we conclude that there are not outliers at the threshold $\alpha=5\%$.

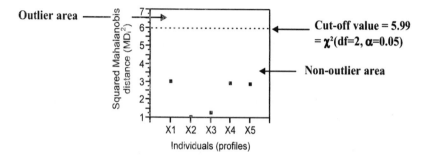

Figure 5.7. Graphical representation of Mahalanobis distance by reference to a Chi-2 cut-off value with $(p-1)$ degree of freedom.

This first part illustrated how MD is calculated and interpreted in order to detect outliers. However, the standard MD suffers from the fact that it is very sensitive to the presence of outliers in the sense that extreme observations (or groups of observations) departing from the main data structure can have a great influence on this distance measure (Rousseeuw and Van Zomeren, 1990). This is somewhat unclear because MD should be able to detect outliers, but the same outliers can heavily affect MD; the reason is the sensitivity of arithmetic mean and covariance matrix to outliers (Hampel et al., 1986): the individual X_i contributes to the calculation of the mean, then this mean will be subtracted from X_i to calculate its MD. Consequently, the standard Mahalanobis distance MD_i can be biased, the outlier X_i can be masked and other points can appear more outlying than they really are. This can be illustrated by the individual X_1 which has an atypically high value for the variable M_3 ($M_3=20$) (Figure 5.8a, b), but which was not detected as outlier. Moreover, scatter plots of variables M_3 vs M_1 and M_2 showed that individual X_1 corresponds to a relationship outlier (Figure 5.8a) analogous to that of point c in Figure 5.5.

A solution consists in inserting more robust mean and covariance estimators in Eqs. 5.2 and 5.4 by using the Jackknife technique (§ VI.2).

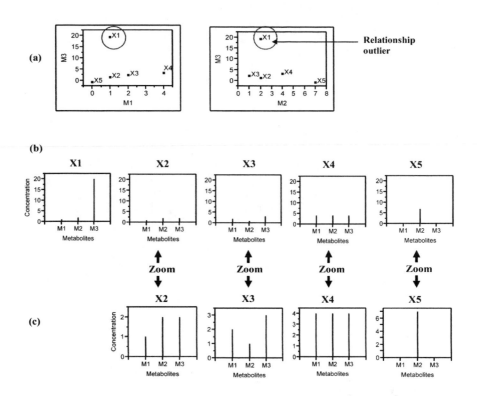

Figure 5.8. (a) Scatter plots between different variables showing a relationship-outlier because of atypically high coordinate for one variable M_3 and ordinary coordinates for the other variables M_1, M_2. (b, c) Concentration profiles of the five analysed profiles X_1-X_5 characterized by three metabolites M_1-M_3.

VI.2. Jackknifed Mahalanobis Distance Computation

Jackknife technique consists in computing, for each multivariate observation x_i, the distance MD_{Ji} from a mean vector and a covariance matrix which were estimated without the observation x_i. This avoids the mean and covariance to be influenced by the values of profile i. In fact, a profile i with a high value can be more easily detected as far from the centroid if it did not contribute to the calculation of mean. Consequently, any multivariate observation x_i characterized by an atypical value x_{ij} can be more easily detected as far from the centroid and/or as discordant by reference to the multivariate distribution of the whole dataset X (Figure 5.9).

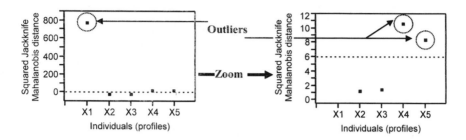

Figure 5.9. Outlier detection based on Mahalanobis distance calculated by the Jackknife technique.

The powerful of Jackknife technique can be illustrated by its ability to detect individual X_1 as outlier because of its extreme value for the variable M_3 resulting in a distorted profile compared to the four other profiles (Figure 5.8b). Moreover, individuals X_4 and X_5 were detected as outliers although their values had comparable levels to those of most of the profiles (Figure 5.8b). The fact that X_4 and X_5 are detected as outliers is not due to the levels of their values but to atypical combinations of the three values (M_1, M_2, M_3) resulting in atypical profiles (Figure 5.8c): X_4 had uniform profile because of equal values for the three variables, whereas X_5 showed a single needle profile because of the null values of the variable M_1 and M_3. Atypical states of profiles X_4 and X_5 seem to be due to uniform shape of X4 and exclusive peak (only one metabolite present) in X5.

VI. 3. Identification of Extreme Profiles by Correspondence Analysis

VI.3.1. General Concepts of Correspondence Analysis

Correspondence analysis (CA) is a multivariate method that can be applied on a data matrix having both additive rows and columns. It aims at analysis of the strongest associations between individuals (rows) (e.g. metabolic profiles) and variables (columns) (e.g. metabolites). On this basis, individuals strongly associated with some variables can be characterized by original or extreme profiles compared to the whole population. In this case, a strong association between an individual and a variable can be identified by a high value of variable j in individual i compared to all the values (Figure 5.10):

- of the other variables ($\neq j$) in the same individual i on the hand, and
- for the same variable j in all the other individuals ($\neq i$) on the other hand.

In other words, CA considers each value not by its absolute but by its relative level both along its row and column (Figure 5.10): for example, in individuals X_3 and X_4, the absolute values (concentration) of variable M_3 (metabolite M_3) are equal to 3 and 4, respectively, leading to consider the second as more important than the first one. However, in terms of relative values, 3 in X_3 and 4 in X_4 represent 50% and 33%, respectively, of the total ofrespective profiles; consequently, the value 3 of profile X_3 is relatively more important than the value 4 in profile X_4, leading to consider individual X_3 as more associated than X_4 to variable M_3. However, by considering all the individuals X_1 to X_5, the relative level 50% of $M_3=3$ in its profile appears to be lower than that $M_3=20$ in X_1 (87%). Finally, individual X_1 appears as the most associated to variable M_3 by considering all the rows (profiles) and columns (variables) of the dataset. To conclude on the outlier or non-outlier state of X_1, all the individuals X_i of the dataset must be considered according to all the variables; this allows to check if X_1 is alone to be extreme (a), or if other individuals are also original under other characteristics (b). In the first case (a), the rarity of X_1 makes to consider it as atypical; in the second case (b), one talks about different trends in the dataset rather than atypical cases (or outliers) (Figure 5.11).

VI.3.2. Basic Computations in Correspondence Analysis

Correspondence analysis (CA) is an exploratory multivariate method which analyses the relative variations within a simple two-way table X (n rows × p columns) containing measures of correspondence between rows and columns. The matrix X consists of additive data both along the rows and columns (e.g. contingency table, concentration dataset, or any homogeneous unit matrix). On this basis, simultaneous or dual analysis of row and column profiles are advantageously possible in CA.

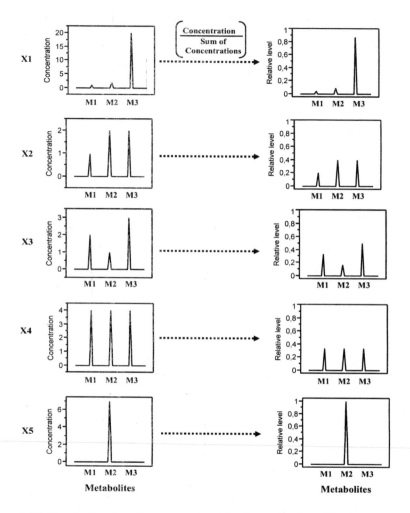

Figure 5.10. Standardization of concentration (absolute values) profiles into relative levels leading to data homogenization at a scale varying between 0 and 1.

Row and column profiles are obtained by dividing each value x_{ij} (e.g. concentration of metabolite j in subject i) by its row and column sums, x_{i+} and x_{+j} respectively:

$$f_i = \frac{x_{ij}}{\sum\limits_{j=1}^{p} x_{ij}} = \frac{x_{ij}}{x_{i+}} \ (j{=}1 \text{ to } p) \qquad f_j = \frac{x_{ij}}{\sum\limits_{i=1}^{n} x_{ij}} = \frac{x_{ij}}{x_{+j}} \ (i{=}1 \text{ to } n) \qquad (5.5)$$

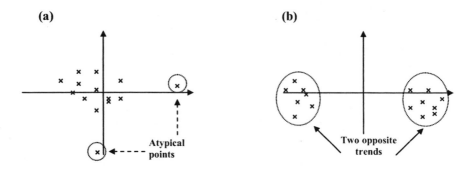

Figure 5.11. Illustration of two dataset structures corresponding to the presence of isolated atypical individual cases (a) and to grouped individuals into well distinct trends (b).

This transformation is appropriate to highlight the strongest associations between rows and columns: two row profiles are more similar if they show comparable relative values for the same column-variables. Reciprocally, two variables will have similar variation trends if their relative values vary in the same way in all the rows. Finally, a row i is strongly associated with a column j if it has a high value x_{ij} for this column compared with all the values of the same row i and of the same column j. This duality along rows and columns requires standardization of each value x_{ij} by the square root of the product of

x_{i+} and x_{+j}: $\sqrt{\dfrac{x_{ij}}{x_{i+}.x_{+j}}}$ (Figure 5.12).

From the matrix T of the standardized values, two analyses are performed to calculate new coordinates (called factorial coordinates) for rows (individuals) and columns (variables), respectively (Figure 5.12). Row analysis is performed on the matrix $T'T$, whereas column analysis is performed on the matrix TT'. One obtains two squared matrices TT' and $T'T$ which have $(p-1)$ eigenvalues λ_j comprised between 0 and 1; p being the smallest dimension of the dataset (generally, in a dataset $(n \times p)$, there are less variables than individuals, i.e. $p<n$). Extreme eigenvalues equal to 0 or 1 are not considered because they correspond to trivial values.

The $(p-1)$ decreasing eigenvalues λ_j are combined with the matrices $T'T$ on the hand and TT' on the other hand, to calculate $(p-1)$ eigenvectors V_j for the rows and for the columns, respectively. Finally, the factorial coordinates of the rows and columns are calculated from the scalar products of eigenvectors v_j by:

- the row profiles (x_{ij}/x_{i+}) weighted by the root square of the respective ratios x_{++}/x_{+j} (row analysis, figure 5.12),
- the column profiles (x_{ij}/x_{+j}) weighted by the the root square of the respective ratios x_{++}/x_{i+} (column analysis, figure 5.12).

The new coordinates resulting from row and column analyses have the characteristic to condense the variability of the initial dataset within a small dimension space $(<p)$ based on independent directions (called factors). The factors have also the property to be successively shorter because they correspond to decreasing eigenvalues; this makes possible to describe the variability of the initial dataset by a minimal dimension space represented by the first factors (Escofier and Pagès, 1991): the first factor (F_1) describes the maximal part of total variability followed be the second (F_2) which describes a maximal part of the remaining variability not described by F_1, etc. . This leads the variability of the dataset to be rapidly condensed into a small dimension space. This is particularly useful in the case of large datasets, what is generally the case in metabolomics.

The computations of factorial coordinates are illustrated by a numerical example based on the previous dataset (Figure 5.6) (Figures 5.13, 5.14). After the calculation of factorial coordinates of the rows along each factor, their sign must correspond to those of the coordinates of the eigenvectors for the columns: for instance, along F_1, the eigenvector of column is V_1 with five coordinates (0.58, -0.12, 0.07, -0.17, -0.78) (Figure 5.14); the calculation of factorial coordinates of the five rows along F_1 gives (-0.59, 0.27, -0.14, 0.24, 1.44) (Figure 5.13) (not shown) ; as the two sets have opposite signs, it is needed to multiply one of them by -1 to obtain appropriate superimposition between rows and columns: Thus F_1 becomes F_1(0.59, -0.27, 0.14, -0.24, -1.44) (Figure 5.13). According to the dataset, such sign correction can or can't occur.

To measure the remoteness between two row-profiles or two column-profiles, CA uses the chi-square distance. The distance between two row profiles i and i' is given by (Escofier and Pagès, 1991; Greenacre, 1984; 1993):

$$d^2(i,i') = \sum_{j=1}^{p} \frac{x_{++}}{x_{+j}} \left(\frac{x_{ij}}{x_{i+}} - \frac{x_{i'j}}{x_{i'+}} \right)^2 \qquad (5.6)$$

where x_{++} is the sum of the whole database, x_{i+}, $x_{i'+}$ are the sums of rows i and i', respectively, and x_{+j} is the sum of column j.

This distance is low when the profiles show similar relative values of several variables, independently of their absolute values (Figure 1.3). Similarly, the distance between two column profiles (e.g. two metabolite variables) j and j' is given by:

$$d^2(j,j') = \sum_{i=1}^{n} \frac{x_{++}}{x_{i+}} \left(\frac{x_{ij}}{x_{+j}} - \frac{x_{ij'}}{x_{+j'}} \right)^2 \qquad (5.7)$$

VI.3.3. Graphical Interpretation of CA Results and Diagnostic of Extreme Profiles

Graphical visualization of the factorial coordinates of rows helps to see how much each individual tends to be extreme or ordinary within the population. At the same time, the scatter plots of factorial coordinates of columns help to identify what and how variables are associated to extreme individuals: an individual i projecting close to a variable j means a high value in individual i for variable j compared with all the individuals and variables of the dataset. Graphically, extreme individual profiles can be highlighted by extreme points along the factors (axes) of CA (Greenacre, 1984, 1993). Moreover, based on the duality in CA, the variables responsible of the extreme states of such individuals are identified as variable-points located in the same projection subspace than corresponding individual-points.

From the numerical example (Figure 5.13), the individuals X_1 and X_5 showed opposite and extreme projections along F_1 (first factor). Moreover, along F_1, the variables M_3 and M_2 projected in the same subspaces than X_1 and X_5, respectively (Figure 5.14); this indicates that the individuals X_1 and X_5 have relatively high values of M_3 and M_2, respectively, by comparison with all the values of the corresponding row and column profiles: in fact, the values $M_3=20$ in X_1 and $M_2=7$ in X_5 represent high maxima both along their rows and columns. The opposition between X_1 and X_5 can be explained by an inverse variability of M_2 and M_3 in X_1 and X_5: X_1 has a high M_3 and a low M_2, whereas X_5 shows inverse characteristics. Moreover, the case (X_5, M_2) appears more extreme along F_1 than (X_1, M_3). This is due to the fact that the value 7 of M_2 in X_5 is relatively more important than the value 20 of M_3 in X_1: 100% versus 87% (Figure 5.10).

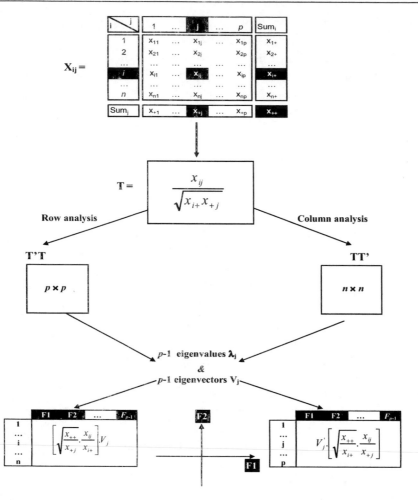

Figure 5.12. Principle of computation of factorial coordinates in correspondence analysis.

Along F_2, the individuals X_3 and X_4 tend to form a group (Figure 5.13) characterized by the variable M_1 (Figure 5.14). This provides information on the presence of a third trend within the dataset. This trend emerges by the fact that the values of $M_1=2$ in X_3 and $M_1=4$ in X_4 are relatively more important than the other values ($0 \leq \leq 4$) both of the rows X_3, X_4 and column M_1. Taking into account the facts that F_2 represents less variability than F_1, the third trend defined by metabolite M_1 in profiles X_3 and X_4 is less extreme than the trends defined by M_3 in X_1 or M_2 in X_5.

Finally, the profile X_2 can be considered as the most ordinary because it projects around the centre of the plane F_1F_2 (Figure 5.13). The same factorial plane of variables shows that such a profile doesn't favor a particular metabolite, although it tends to be more close to the profiles X_3, X_4, i.e. to the third trend (along F_2).

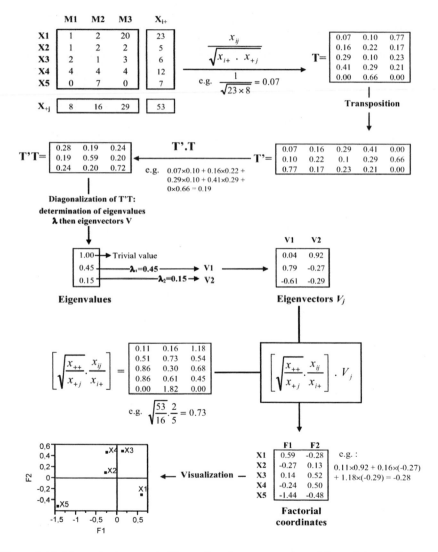

Figure 5.13. Numerical example illustrating the computation of factorial coordinates of rows in correspondence analysis (row analysis).

Moreover, X_3 and X_4 appear to be opposite to X_1 and X_5 along F_2 which is defined by variable M_1 (Figures 5.13, 5.14). This can be explained by the fact that M_1 has relatively high values in X_3, X_4 against relatively low (minimal) values in X_1 and X_5.

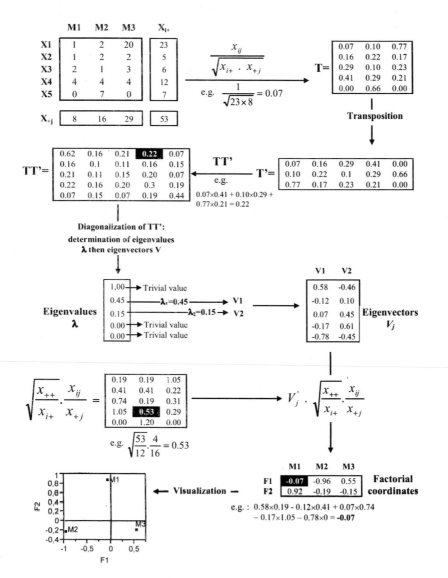

Figure 5.14. Numerical example illustrating the computation of factorial coordinates of columns in correspondence analysis (column analysis).

VI.4. Outlier Diagnostic Based on Andrews Curves

VI.4.1. General Concepts

Andrews curves represent a strong graphical tool to analyze the homogeneity and diversity of profiles from a multivariate dataset under the Euclidean distance criterion. They provide a plane representation of the multivariate distribution of the profiles based on a Fourier transformation: each individual (profile) is represented by a sine-cosine curve calculated from its initial coordinates at different rotation angles α. The relative positions of Andrews curves provide condensate information on differences/remoteness between corresponding individuals under the Euclidean criterion. Outlier individuals can be identified by their Andrews curves isolated from the rest of the curves at a given rotation angle.

VI.4.2. Computation of Andrews Curves

The measured values of the p variables in a given profile are used into a sine-cosine function to calculate a serial of values corresponding to several rotation angles α ($-\pi \leq \alpha \leq \pi$) (Figure 5.15a). The sine-cosine function $f_i(\alpha)$ calculated for profile i at a rotation angle α has the form:

$$f_i(\alpha) = \frac{x_{i1}}{\sqrt{2}} + x_{i2} \sin(\alpha) + x_{i3} \cos(\alpha) + x_{i4} \sin(2\alpha) + x_{i5} \cos(2\alpha) + ... \quad (5.8)$$

By using q different α values, one obtains a set of q coordinates $f_i(\alpha)$ from which the Andrews curve of individual i can be plotted as $f_i(\alpha)$ versus α (Seber, 1984; Everitt and Dunn, 1992) (Figure 5.15b).

VI.4.3. Graphical Outlier Diagnostic Based on Andrews Curves

By plotting the Andrews curves of all the individuals, one can expect to see isolated bands of curves representing outlying individuals, which separate from the compact mass of curves representing the homogeneous population (Figure 5.15b). The distances between Andrews curves are proportional to the Euclidean distances between corresponding individuals.

A drawback of this method is that an interchange of variables leads to a different picture. However, this is not problematic in case of kinetic (concentration-time) datasets where the concentration data are ordered in time and cannot be interchanged.

Application of Andrews curves to the previous dataset (Figure 5.15) shows a central zone containing condensed curves from which other curves separate gradually leading to some extreme cases: the most isolated curve is that of profile X_1; it is followed by the curve of X_5 then X_4 which show only a slight separation from the compact centre containing the ordinary profiles X_2 and X_3. The profiles X_1, X_5 and X_4 are particularly characterized by the highest values in the dataset leading to their more or less outlying states. Under the Euclidean concept, X_1 shows the most atypical state because it has the highest value ($M_3=20$) compared to the significantly lower values of the dataset.

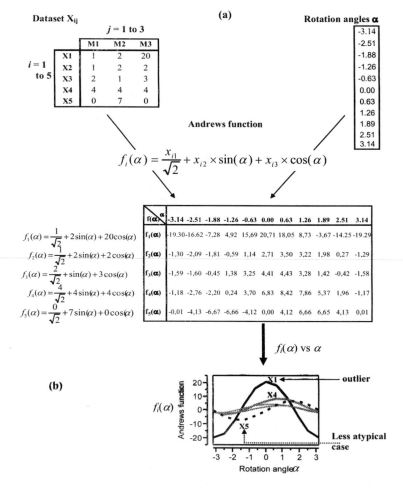

Figure 5.15. Numerical example illustrating computation of Andrews curves and their graphical representation and interpretation.

Chapter 6

WEIGHTED METABOLIC
PROFILES ANALYSIS

I. GENERAL CONCEPTS AND AIM

Metabolic systems are characterized by high chemical polymorphisms that can be highlighted by high variability of metabolic profiles leading to the apparition of different extreme trends. Such metabolic trends (MbTrs) are characterized by high regulations for some metabolites compared to all the others. Extreme profiles representing MbTrs can be statistically identified by means of correspondence analysis (CA) (Chapter 5, VI.3) followed by a cluster analysis such as HCA (Chapter 4):

MbTrs in a given population (system) can be highlighted by CA which is able to extract extreme profiles showing extreme regulations for some metabolites. Then, the results of CA will be used by HCA to classify all the profiles of the studied population into clusters representing the different identified MbTrs (Figure 6.1a) (Semmar et al., 2007). Such a statistical classification is justified by the fact that any intermediate profile is more or less close to a given MbTr. Moreover, the extreme profiles are not isolated from the intermediate ones because the set of all profiles issued from a same metabolic system show generally gradual variations leading to a continuum topology. After a typological stratification of such a continuum into different clusters (MbTrs), each cluster will contain:

-   Extreme profile defining the fingerprint of corresponding MbTr.

- Less extreme or intermediate profiles providing intrinsic variability within the MbTr.

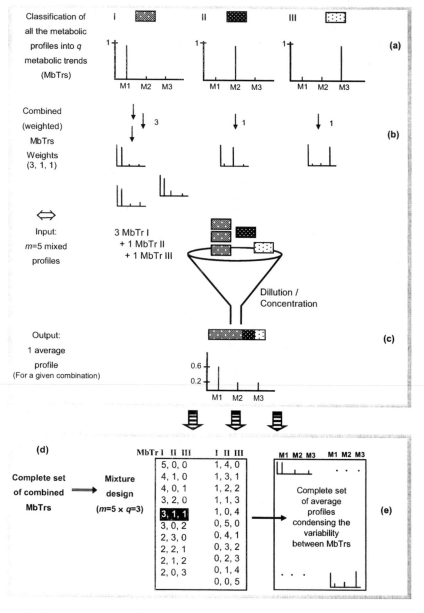

Figure 6.1. Basic concepts and steps of weighted metabolic profiles analysis (WMPA) (Semmar, 2010).

From the whole metabolic variability structured into clusters representing well defined MbTrs, the basic principles of weighted metabolic profiles analysis (WMPA) are established around the following question: what functional processes are behind the gradual variations in metabolic profiles leading to the emergence of the different MbTrs? Such a question can be statistically approached by combining the variabilities of the different clusters representing the different MbTrs. A given combination is a mixture operation in which the different MbTrs have well defined weights (Figure 6.1b). In other words, all the combinations differ ones from the others by the weights that they attribute to the different MbTrs (Figure 6.1d). Such weights vary by the occurrence levels of profiles representing the different MbTrs. Therefore, the mixed profiles will contribute to reinforce or attenuate the fingerprint of each MbTrs according to the different weights of such MbTrs (i.e; relative occurrences of representative profiles in the mixture). Such a mixing is analogous to concentration/dilution processes the effect of which can be summarized by the average profile of all the individual profiles representing the different weighted MbTrs (Figure 6.1c). Iterations of such combinations set and resulting average profiles are needed to obtain results taking into account the whole variability of profiles in the different MbTrs. After several iterations, the complete set of average profiles resulting from the different combinations is expected to bring simulated information on gradual metabolic variability due to changes in weighting of the different MbTrs. Therefore, such variability can be analysed to extract a backbone picture on the variability of the central metabolic machine governing the emergence of the different MbTrs (Figure 6.1e). For that, from the average profiles dataset (resulting from iterated combinations design), relationships between metabolites will be graphically analysed to understand metabolic regulations responsible for the observed chemical polymorphism. Thus, WMPA represents a useful approach to analyse the metabolic origins of chemical polymorphisms in biological populations (Semmar et al., 2007; Semmar, 2010).

II. METHODOLOGY

To analyse functional aspect of a metabolic system from the set of its regulation profiles, WMPA carries out a complete set of combinations between such profiles classified *a priori* into different MbTrs. Such combinations attribute gradual weights to the different MbTrs favoring to cover the space of all the gradual variations between them. Then, such a space can be graphically explored to identify regulation ways between metabolites leading to the development of different MbTrs.

Starting from a dataset of n metabolic profiles containing p metabolites, six methodological steps are applied in WMPA to analyse the functional relationships between metabolites having led to a chemical polymorphism consisting of q MbTrs (Figures 6.2, 6.3):

i.   Classification of the n profiles into the q well defined MbTrs by applying a HCA on the ordination results given by CA (Figure 6.2a).

ii. Combinations of the metabolic profiles according to a mixture design attributing gradual weights to each of the q MbTrs (Figure 6.2b).

iii. From each combination, an average profile is calculated as elementary response representing the q weighted MbTrs (Figure 6.2c).

iv. Iteration of the mixture design to take into account the variability of profiles within each MbTr (Figure 6.3a). The k iterations lead to cumulate k responses from each combination (Figure 6.3b).

v.   Calculation of final (smoothed) response matrix by averaging the k iterated elementary response matrices (Figure 6.3c).

vi. Graphical analysis of relationships between metabolites from the final response matrix containing a complete set of smoothed profiles (Figure 6.3d).

II.1. Classification of Metabolic Profiles into Metabolic Trends

Starting from a dataset (n profiles $\times p$ metabolites), CA is initially applied to analyse the metabolic variability of the system in terms of different extreme trends defined by extreme regulations for some metabolites. CA structures the whole variability of the system into p-1 factors representing decreasing and complementary variability parts (Chapter 5, VI.3). Among the p-1 factors, the r first ones have the advantage to condensate the main variability of the system, and they will be separated from the p-1-r remaining factors which contain some local or residual variabilities. From the r first factors of CA, one supposes that q MbTrs were identified (Chapter 5, VI.3.3). On the r first factors (i.e. the r first factorial coordinates of the n individuals), a HCA can be applied to classify the n individual profiles into q MbTrs.

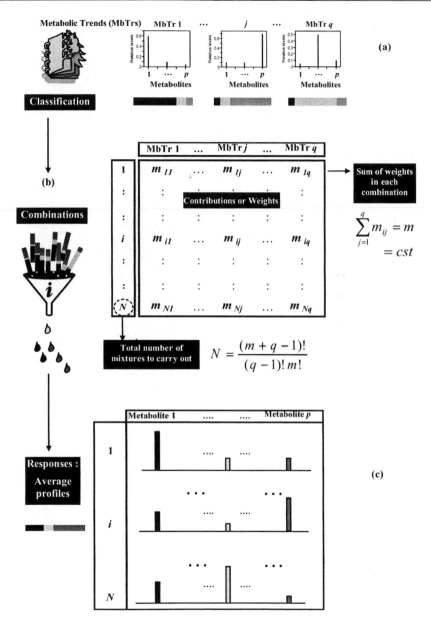

Figure 6.2. The three first steps (a-c) (among six) of weighted metabolic profiles analysis. Calculation of elementary response matrix containing average profiles (c) from a complete set of combinations between metabolic profiles (b) representing q metabolic trends (MbTrs) *a priori* classified (a).

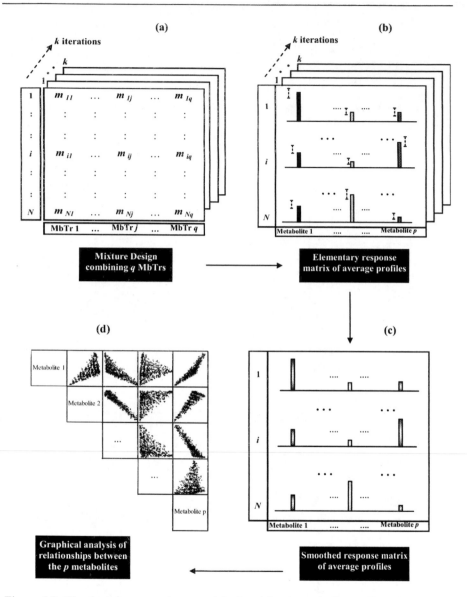

Figure 6.3. The three last steps (among six) of weighted metabolic profiles analysis. Iteration of the mixture design and its response matrix (step 4) (a, b) leading to calculate a final smoothed matrix of average profiles (step 5) (c) from which relationships between metabolites can be graphically analysed (step 6) (d).

II.2. Description of Mixture Design to Metabolic Profiles combinations

Starting from q clusters of metabolic profiles representing q well defined MbTrs, a complete set of combinations between such q components will be applied to generate a space of gradual variations between them (Figure 6.4). This set of combinations can be applied on the basis of a mixture design called Scheffé's matrix (Figure 6.4c): In this design, the q MbTrs (q components to mix) are represented into q columns and their different mixtures in rows.

Combinations between the q MbTrs are carried out by mixing a constant number m of metabolic profiles representing such MbTrs. The different mixtures differ by the presence levels m_j that they attribute to the different MbTrs j ($\sum_{j=1}^{q} m_j = m$). In other words, in a given mixture, each MbTr j has a weight m_j/m varying between 0 (if $m_j=0$) and 1 (if $m_j=m$). For instance, if $m=10$ and $q=4$, each mixture of Scheffé's matrix will contain 10 profiles belonging to the 4 MbTrs according to four different presence levels m_j (e.g. $m_1=2$, $m_2=4$, $m_3=1$, $m_4=3$; $\sum_{j=1}^{q=4} m_j = 10 = m$) (Figures 6.4c, 6.2b).

From the number q of components (MbTrs) to combine and the total number m of elements (profiles) per combination (per mixture), the total number of mixtures needed to be carried out is given by the formula (Figure 6.2b):

$$N = \frac{(m+q-1)!}{(q-1)!m!} \tag{6.1}$$

N corresponds to the number of rows of Scheffé's matrix from which the space of gradual variations between the q components (MbTrs) can be generated. With $m=10$ and $q=2, 3, 4$, it results three Scheffé's matrices having 11, 66 and 286 mixtures (rows), respectively (Figure 6.5a).

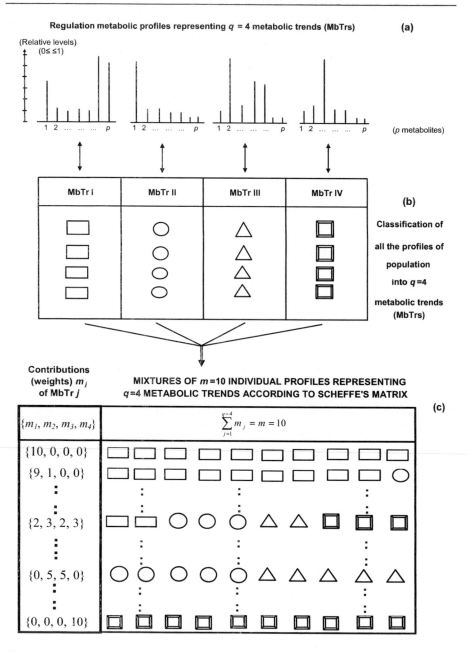

Figure 6.4. Illustration of a Scheffé's matrix (c) combining $m=10$ variable elements (e.g. metabolic profiles) representing $q=4$ components (e.g. metabolic trends) (a, b).

Geometrically, the N mixtures combining the q components define a simplex space with $(q\text{-}1)$ dimensions: thus for $q=2$, 3, 4 components, the simplex space is a segment, equilateral triangle and tetrahedron, respectively (Figure 6.5b) (Semmar, 2010; Duineveld et al., 1993a, b). Such simplex geometries defined by weighting constraints (regulations, concentrations/dillutions) show some analogies with convex cones defined by flux irreversibility and capacity constraints (Figure 2.3).

II.3. Application of Mixture Design Based on Random Sampling Rules

Simplex mixture design is applied to analyse regulation processes between metabolites which would be at the origin of observed chemical polymorphism. The concept of metabolic regulation is initially based on the decomposition of a whole unit into different parts which will be distributed between different components of system (e.g. metabolites, metabolic pathways, etc.).

At metabolite scale, metabolic regulation can be assessed by dividing the concentration of each metabolite by the sum of concentrations of all the metabolites belonging to a same profile (Figure 1.3). Thus, the concentrations are initially converted into relative levels to obtain regulation profiles.

Beyond metabolite and metabolic pathway, a metabolic profile can be conceived as a high-scale variability unit providing a whole picture on functional regulations of metabolic system. By considering profile as variability basis, any profile of metabolic system can be translated in terms of combination between MbTrs associated to different weights. Such weights govern the output profile which will tend more or less to the corresponding MbTrs (Figure 6.1c).

A complete set of combinations between MbTrs is expected to translate the effects of gradual expressions of such MbTrs on variability of the metabolic system. Two variabilities need to be considered viz., between and within MbTrs. The first is directly covered by the complete set of combinations given by Scheffé's matrix (Figure 6.2b); the second requires iterations of Scheffé's mixture design leading to repeat the combinations by considering the variability of profiles within each MbTr (Figure 6.3a). The double operation consisting in applying and iterating the mixture design can be summarized by two bootstrapping operations from which the variabilities between and within MbTrs will be progressively extracted (Figure 6.6).

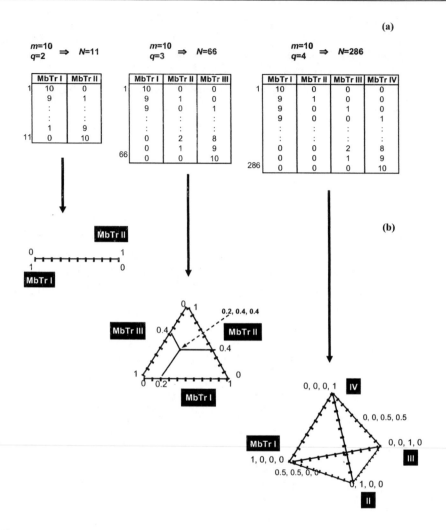

Figure 6.5. Different Scheffé' matrices (a) and corresponding simplex spaces (b).

II.3.1. Bootstrapping between Metabolic Trends
and Corresponding Response

Bootstrapping between MbTrs consists simply of the application of all the mixtures given by Scheffé's matrix according to random sampling rules:

Each mixture of Scheffé's matrix is performed by randomly sampling m profiles from the q MbTrs j. By fixing the number m, we have to carry out N mixtures between the q MbTrs (j) by varying their contributions m_j the ones at the expense of the others: $\sum_{j=1}^{q} m_j = m$. The N randomly sampled mixtures corresponding to N different combinations between MbTrs, can be simply considered as a bootstrapping between MbTrs (Figures 6.6a, 6.7a).

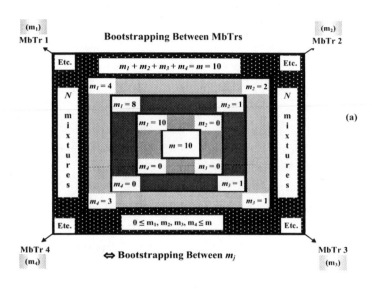

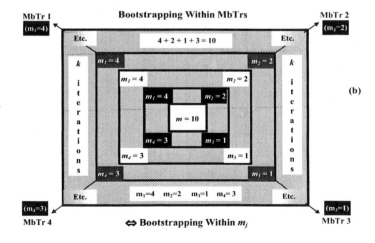

Figure 6.6. Double bootstrapping applied in weighted metabolic profile analysis to extract variabilities between (a) and within (b) metabolic trends (MbTrs). m_j: weights of the different MbTrs j contributing to a total weight m (here, fixed to $m=10$).

To evaluate what metabolic profile could be expected from each mixture of weighted MbTrs, an average profile is calculated from the m individual profiles of such a mixture (Figure 6.7b):

$$\overline{y} = \frac{\sum\limits_{j=1}^{q}\sum\limits_{e=1}^{m_j} y_{ej}}{m} \tag{6.2}$$

Where:

y_{ej}: value (relative level) of the considered metabolite in the profile e of the MbTr j.

q: total number of MbTrs.

m_j: number of profiles or the weight of MbTr j.

m: total number of profiles in any mixture.

In an average profile representing a mixture i, the relative level $\overline{y}$ of a given metabolite increases with the weight m_j of its highest regulation MbTr j. For a given mixture $(m_1,..,m_j,..,m_q)$, the m_j values representing the m_j profiles of each MbTr j will be diluted or concentrated according to the relative importance of m_j (Figure 1.10).

In total, N average profiles will be calculated and stored into the elementary response matrix R_E (Figure 6.7b).

II.3.2. Bootstrapping Within Metabolic Trends and Corresponding Response

At the previous step where a single mixture design was applied, each of the N average profiles was obtained from only m randomly sampled individuals, whereas the whole population contains much more than m individuals. This results in important under-estimation of the variability within each MbTr. As consequence of such under-estimation, the elementary response matrix R_E will give non-stable (non-reliable) picture on the metabolic variability of the system. To obtain a reliable picture on the metabolic variability, iterations of the mixture design are needed: by applying K iterations, the m profiles of each mixture are randomly sampled K times (Figure 6.6b). The K iterated samplings increase the diversity of profiles contributing to each of the N mixtures (Figure 6.7c): After the K iterations, each combination $(m_1, \ldots, m_q)$ between the q MbTrs, will be represented by K sets $(m_1, \ldots, m_q)$ of m newly randomly sampled profiles. Thus, the K sets of the m_j profiles belonging to a same MbTr j will bring information on the variability within such MbTr. Under a technic aspect, such K iterated random samplings consist of a bootstrapping within MbTrs (Figure 6.6b).

From the K iterations of the mixture design, K elementary response matrices containing N average profiles will be obtained covering variability between and within MbTrs (Figure 6.7c). Finally, a reliable picture on the variability of metabolic system can be obtained by calculating a final smoothed response matrix R_F from the average of the K iterated elementary response matrices (Figure 6.7d):

$$\overline{\overline{y}}_i = \frac{\sum_{k=1}^{K} \overline{y}_{ik}}{K} \qquad (6.3)$$

Where:

$\overline{\overline{y}}_i$: final average of mixture i calculated from the K elementary averages $\overline{y}_{ik}$ calculated separately on each iteration k of such mixture.

k: index of iterations

K: total number of iterations (= 50 in figure 6.7)

II.4. Graphical Analysis of Smoothed Results Issued from Iterated Simplex Mixture design

The smoothed matrix contains N final average metabolic profiles (rows) with p metabolites (columns) the relative levels of which vary gradually. From this response matrix, the variations between metabolites can be graphically visualized by means of scatter plots. Such variations will be characterized by different directions, extents and shapes helping to interpret the intrinsic variability of the metabolic system. In the mixture design, such a variability was progressively incorporated, filtered and smoothed during the iterated averaging resulting from the double bootstrapping (between and within MbTrs). Geometrically, such iterated averaging constraints the simplex space to rotations and compressions under the effects of variation ranges and variation types of the initial data (Duineveld et al., 1993a).

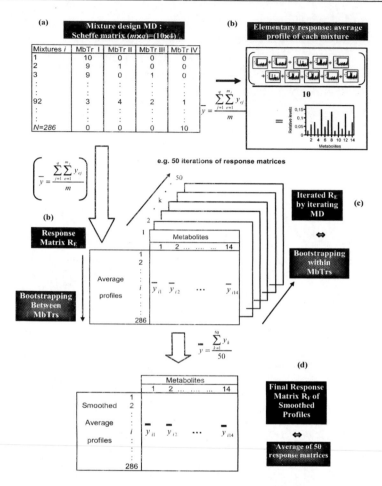

Figure 6.7. Illustration of bootstrapping in WMPA applied to a mixture design (m=10 $\times$ q=4), i.e. combining m=10 profiles (of 14 metabolites) representing q=4 MbTrs.

Relationships between metabolites highlighted by the scatter plots of smoothed matrix R_F (N average profiles $\times$ p metabolites) can be classified into three types (Figure 6.8): (a) thin inclined, (b) scale-dependent, (c) MbTr-dependent multidirectional relationships:

1. Thin inclinations indicate global relationships between metabolites at the scale of the whole metabolic system where the different MbTrs have variable expression degrees. In other words, a thin global relationship between two metabolites translates a stable or permanent expression in despite of the variations of all the other metabolites.

Positive global relationships can concern metabolites belonging to a precursor-product metabolic chain; negative global relationships can concern metabolites belonging to competitive metabolic pathways (Figure 6.8a).

2. Scale-dependent relationships consist of a global trend containing several local or systematic variations which regularly arise (Figure 6.8b). Such double-scale relationships indicate metabolites having two types of relationships at once: the global trend can be interpreted as a relationship between the two concerned metabolites at the scale of the whole metabolic system, i.e. taking into account the variations of all the other metabolites. Local or systematic variations can be indicative of a relationship restricted to the subspace defined by the two concerned metabolites disregarding all the other metabolites (Figure 6.9b). A local relationship can have a correlation sign opposite to that of the global trend which includes it. For example, two competitive metabolites belonging to a same metabolic pathway can manifest positive global and negative local correlations: positive global correlation means that the two metabolites sustain a common metabolic pathway against other pathways; negative local correlation reveals their competitivity within their common pathway (e.g. for a precursor or enzyme) (Semmar et al., 2007).

3. MbTr-dependent multidirectional relationships are graphically identified from non-compressed and non-oriented simplex clouds indicating relationships with large variability and multiple trends (Figure 6.8c). Such cases can be interpreted as flexible relationships between metabolites depending on the considered metabolic trend. For a given MbTr, a characteristic functional trajectory within the scatter plot can be highlighted taking into account the $(m+1)$ weights m_j (0 to m) of such a MbTr: each point of the simplex cloud is originated from a combination between the q MbTrs where the considered MbTr j has a weight m_j (m being constant, the weight m_j/m depends only on m_j; therefore, one will use m_j instead of m_j/m). Taking into account the N points of the simplex space, the projection of the $(m+1)$ weights of the considered MbTr on the N corresponding points leads to define a weight distribution in such a space. Therefore, the points corresponding to a same weight can be graphically located by a confidence ellipse (e.g. 95%). Finally, the spatial chaining of $(m+1)$ confidence ellipses (from weight 0 to weight m) highlight a trajectory (from 0 to m) along which the emergence of considered

MbTr can be drawn (Figure 6.8c): the weight m corresponds to a full development of corresponding MbTr, whereas the weight 0 means its absence (non-functionality or silence). The trajectory linking the ellipse of weight 0 to that of weight m will be analysed to understand how the two considered metabolites varied the ones with respect to the other under the development of the considered MbTr. Finally, the q trajectories corresponding to the q MbTrs will help to understand the metabolic flexibility responsible for the observed chemical polymorphism through different regulation ways of metabolites (Semmar et al., 2007; Semmar, 2010).

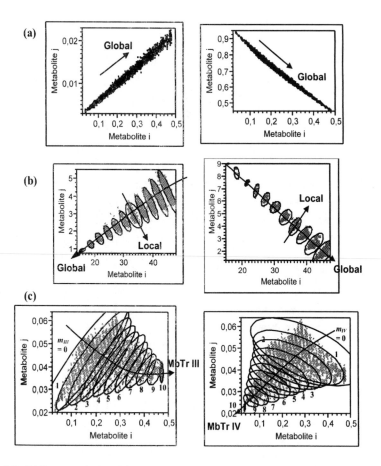

Figure 6.8. Different relationships between metabolites that can be graphically analysed from the smoothed response matrix Rf given by weighted metabolic profile analysis ; (a) global, (b) global and local, (c) metabolic trend-dependent relationships (Semmar et al., 2007; Semmar, 2010).

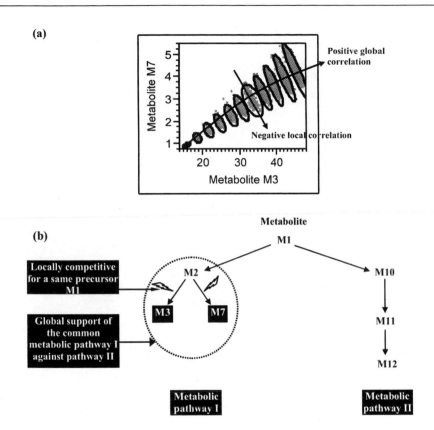

Figure 6.9. (a) Illustration of a correlation locally negative and globally positive correlation; (b) Possible metabolic factor generating such scale dependent correlation, e.g. metabolites M3 and M7 compete each other in metabolic pathway I (negative local correlation) but sustain their common pathway I against the competitive pathway II (positive global correlation).

Chapter 7

TIME-DEPENDENT ANALYSIS OF METABOLIC SYSTEMS

I. BACKGROUND OF DIFFERENT APPROACHES

Metabolic systems can be analysed taking into account their variabilities in time. There are different approaches to analyse the time-dependent variability of metabolic systems, based on different considerations or conceptualisations of time-dependent processes. Deterministic compartment modeling, stochastic-based fitting and dynamic stability analysis represent different approaches (among several others) to analyse the variabilities of systems in time (Ritschel and Kearns, 1999; Holz and Fahr, 2001; Veng-Pedersen, 2001; Anderson et al., 1988; Matis and Wherly, 1985, 1990; Smith et al., 1997; Van Rossum et al., 1989; Heikkilä, 1999). Such analyses include fitting of kinetic curves and computations of associated variability parameters.

Processes governing the kinetic variabilities of metabolic systems can be conceived as successive phases resulting in concentration increase, decrease or stationarity. Such kinetic phases are known in pharmacokinetics under the abbreviation ADME corresponding to Absorption-Distribution-Metabolism-Elimination (Ritschel and Kearns, 1999). They are mathematically formalized by means of deterministic compartment analysis based on system decomposition into different phases (Holz and Fahr, 2001; Ritschel and Kearns, 1999). Increasing phase of concentration can be linked to different processes including biosynthesis, secretion or absorption. Decreasing phase of concentration can result from distribution, storage, transformation (metabolism) or elimination. Stationarity is reached when increase (input) and decrease (output) processes become balanced. Taking into account the variation phases of metabolic system, appropriate deterministic models can be developed to directly predict state variables of system in time (e.g. concentration vs time).

Alternatively to the deterministic approach, stochastic models can be applied to fit directly the shape of a concentration-time curve by means of an appropriate probability density function (pdf) (Matis, 1988; Purdue, 1974, 1979; Matis and Wehrly, 1985, 1990; Matis and Kiffe, 2000, Lansky, 1996; Wimmer et al., 1999; Levine and Hwa, 2007; Matis et al., 1983; Piotrovskii, 1987; Heikkilä, 1999; Weiss, 1983, 1984; Anderson et al., 1988; Beal, 1987). Stochastic models, called also probabilistic models, provide probabilities on the system state instead of direct levels of state variables (e.g. concentrations). Then, the probabilities can be converted into state variables' levels (e.g. concentrations) by a single product of the probability and a total (integrated) value of the state variable. Such a total value is *a priori* intended to fragment (distribute) through the system according a law governed by the appropriate pdf.

Time-dependent processes can be also conceived around the question of the "how does the system behave after a slight perturbation?". After a small perturbation, the system can either return to its equilibrium or evolve away from it. Such a dynamic system response is analysed by considering the simultaneous variations in time of all its parameters (e.g. metabolites) relatively the ones to the others. Mathematical analysis of such variations helps to interpret behavior trajectories of the system including oscillatory (cyclic) and non-oscillatory (translational) processes leading to stable or instable final states. Such analysis is known under the terms of dynamic stability analysis and it is based on the Jacobian matrix calculation (Abraham and Shaw, 1981; Sprott, 2003, Strogatz, 2000; Steuer, 2007).

II. DETERMINISTIC KINETIC ANALYSIS OF METABOLIC SYSTEM BASED ON VARIATION PHASE AND COMPARTMENT CONCEPT

II.1. General Presentation of Different Concentration-Time Scatter Plots

For a given metabolite, temporal variations of concentrations in a biological matrix (e.g. plasma) can be analysed by means of scatter-plots of concentration vs time. Three basic graphical shapes can be generally observed (Figure 7.1):

a.   Strictly decreasing concentration from a maximum value C_0 observed at initial time (Figure 7.1a).
b.   Peak concentration separating initial increasing and final decreasing phases (Figure 7.1b).
c.   Increasing phase leading to a stationarity (Figure 7.1c).

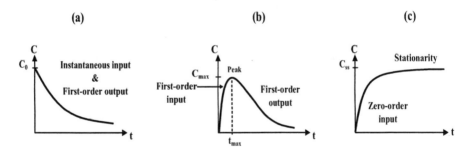

Figure 7.1. different concentration-time curves showing different variation shapes which can be analysed by different kinetic computation and formulations. t: time; C: concentration; C_0: initial concentration; C_{max}: maximal concentration; t_{max}: time of C_{max}; C_{ss}: steady state concentration.

In pharmacology, these three variation shapes can be observed after intraveinous bolus injection (Figure 7.1a), oral or *per os* administration (Figure 7.1b) and continuous infusion or repeated administrations (Figure 7.1c) (Ritschel and Kearns, 1999; Boroujerdi, 2002; Shargel and Yu, 1999). In kinetic modeling, these three cases correspond to instantaneous input with first-order output (a), first-order input and output (b) and zero-order input models. First-order and zero-order mean variation processes which dependent or no on the remaining concentration levels, respectively. Although such models are generally applied to fit the kinetic variations of drugs in humans or animals, they can be used to understand more processes governing evolutions of intrinsic (e.g. hormones) or extrinsic (e.g. dietary) compounds within living bodies (Semmar et al., 2005b; Semmar and Simon, 2006; Hollman et al., 1996).

II.2. Preliminary Graphical Analysis to Compute Kinetic Parameters

The kinetics of a given metabolite (drug) can be described on the basis of different parameters that can be graphically determined from its concentration-time scatter plot:

The first parameter that can be graphically determined is the number of decreasing phases of metabolite: from a maximal value, the metabolite concentration (C) can decrease according to one or more phases. Each decreasing phase is characterized by a frankly distinct slope which can be interpreted in terms of kinetic rate of such a step. As the concentration variation is non-linear (exponential) in time, the different decreasing phases can be more accurately identified from a logarithmic transformation, i.e. from $\ln(C)$ vs time (Figures 7.2, 7.3). In the semi-logarithmic plot, each decreasing linear phase is interpreted as a compartment, i.e. conceptual space through which the metabolite concentration is controlled by distribution, transformation and elimination processes:

When one linear decreasing phase is observed, the metabolite is considered to be simply eliminated from central and unique compartment (Figure 7.2).

(i)   When two linear decreasing phases are observed in time, the first one (faster) is interpreted as a distribution phase revealing the existence of a peripheral compartment in addition to the central one (Figure 7.3). The second decreasing phase is slower and is attributed to elimination process from the central compartment.

(ii) Beyond two decreasing phases, more and more deep compartments can be attributed to metabolite distribution, e.g. plasma (Cpt 1, central) → interstitial space (Cpt 2) → Cytoplasm (Cpt 3) → Orgnelles (Cpt 4) (Ritschel and Kearn, 1999).

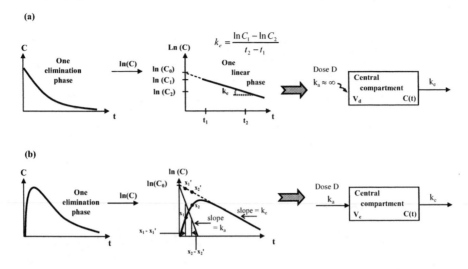

Figure 7.2. Graphical analysis of one decreasing phase kinetics corresponding to one-compartment models. (a) Instantaneous input with first-order output; (b) first-order input and output.

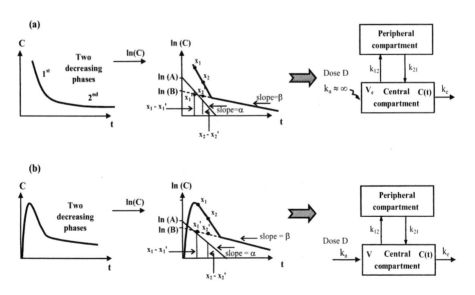

Figure 7.3. Graphical analysis of two decreasing phase kinetics corresponding to two-compartment models. (a) Instantaneous input with first-order output; (b) first-order input and output.

After the number of compartments has been graphically determined, each decreasing phase can be characterized by some rate constants (expressed in time^{-1}) which quantify distribution and elimination rates. Such rate constants are graphically calculated from the slopes of corresponding linear decreasing phases. Analogously, absorption rate can be graphically determined from the initial increasing phase in the case of first-order input model (Figure 7.1b). Calculations of these different rate constants and other metabolic parameters are detailed in the following sections.

II.3. COMPARTMENT MODEL FORMULATIONS

Mathematically, the variation of concentration in time can be modeled by algebraic sum of negative exponential terms representing different increasing and/or decreasing phases highlighted by semi-logarithmic plot. The exponential terms are of the form $C_{tot}e^{-kt}$ where:

- C_{tot} represents the total concentration from which the decrease starts or to which the increase tends.
- k is a rate constant representing increase or decrease process.
- t is the time.

As e^{-kt} is a decreasing function, it will be used to model decreasing processes (e.g. distribution, elimination). Consequently, inverse (increasing) processes (e.g. absorption, secretion, infusion) can be modeled by using the function form $-e^{-kt}$ which is increasing function.

II.3.1. One-Compartment Model with Instantaneous
Input and First-Order Output

This model is applied when the total concentration of a metabolite is observed at initial time ($t=0$), then eliminated into a single decreasing phase (Figure 7.2a). Instantaneous input can be mathematically defined by a Dirac δ-pulse responsible for the whole block-occurrence of total concentration at $t=0$ in the compartment (Holz and Fahr, 2001).

Its formulation is based on the assumption that kinetic variation of (decrease in) concentration (dC/dt) in the (central) compartment (e.g. plasma) is proportional to the concentration $C(t)$ still remaining at time t in that compartment; such a basic assumption derives from Fick's diffusion law and is at the origin of the term "first-order output" (Ritschel and Kearns, 1999; Shargel and Yu, 1999):

$$\frac{dC(t)}{dt} = -k_e \cdot C(t) \tag{7.1}$$

The parameter k_e in Eq. 7.1 represents the elimination rate constant of the metabolite from the central compartment. It corresponds to the slope of the linear elimination phase in the scatter plot ln(Concentration) vs time (Figure 7.2a):

$$k_e = \frac{\ln C_1 - \ln C_2}{t_2 - t_1} \tag{7.2}$$

Analytical disposition function of concentration C(t) can be obtained by integrating Eq. 7.1:

$$\frac{dC(t)}{dt} = -k_e \cdot C(t) \quad \Leftrightarrow \quad \frac{C(t)}{dC(t)} = -k_e dt$$

$$\Rightarrow \ln C(t) = -k_e t + cst$$

$$\Leftrightarrow C(t) = e^{(-k_e t + cst)} = e^{cst} \times e^{-k_e t}$$

$$\Leftrightarrow C(t) = C_0 \cdot e^{-k_e t} = \frac{D}{V_d} \cdot e^{-k_e t} \tag{7.3}$$

With:

C_0: concentration at initial time $t=0$.

D: total amount (or administrated dose) of metabolite (drug) in the central compartment.

V_d: called apparent volume of distribution because it does'nt necessarily refer to any physiologic compartment in the body. It is simply the size of a compartment necessary to account for the total amount of compound (drug) in the body if it was present throughout the body at the same concentration found in the central compartment (plasma). In other words, V_d can be defined as hypothetical volume one would obtain if all of the compound would be in the whole body based on its actual concentration found in blood. The major determinant on Vd is the relative strength of biding of the compound to tissue components as compared with plasma proteins. If a compound (drug) is very

tightly bound by tissues and not by blood, most of the compound in the body
will be held in the tissue and very little in the plasma, so that the drug will
appear to be dissolved in a large volume of distribution V_d. Thus, a higher V_d
indicates more affinity of the compound for tissues (e.g. drug with high lipid
solubility) (Figure 7.4). This can be interpreted from Eq. 7.3 showing that
increase of V_d (in denominator) results in a decrease (dilution) of $C(t)$ in the
central compartment (plasma) (Figure 7.4). Graphically, V_d can be calculated
by the formula (Ritschel and Kearn, 1999; Bouroujerdi, 2002):

$$V_d = \frac{D}{k_e \cdot AUC} \tag{7.4}$$

Where AUC is the area under the concentration-time curve. It can be
calculated by the trapezoid rule (Eq. 7.6):

$$AUC_0^\infty = AUC_0^{t_n} + AUC_{t_n}^\infty \qquad (\mu g/ml).h \tag{7.5}$$

With:

$$AUC_0^{t_n} = \sum_{i=0}^{n} \left(\frac{C_i + C_{i+1}}{2} \right) \left(t_{i+1} - t_i \right) \tag{7.6}$$

And

$$AUC_{t_n}^\infty = \frac{C_n}{k_e} \tag{7.7}$$

In Eq. 7.6, the index i identifies successive concentration measurements: $i=0$
for the initial concentration C_0 measured at time t_0; $i=n$ for the last
concentration C_n (Eq. 7.7) measured at the last time t_n. In Eq. 7.7, k_e is the
elimination rate constant calculated by Eq. 7.2.

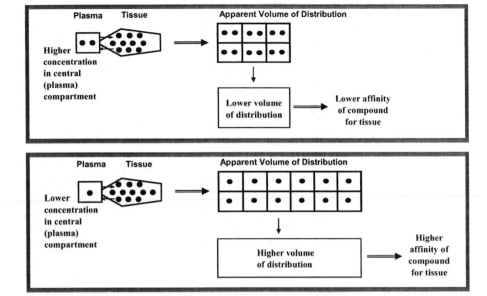

Figure 7.4. Two examples illustrating the hypothetical concept of volume of distribution. A same amount (12 points in all) can be hypothetically distributed in a smaller (6 squares) or a greater (12 squares) space corresponding to lower and higher apparent volume of distribution V_d, respectively.

II.3.2. Two-Compartments Model with Instantaneous Input and First-Order Output

Two-compartments model is used when the concentration decreases according to two successive steps representing fast and slow kinetics, respectively. The variation in concentration due to the succession of such two decreasing phases is mathematically formalized by a sum of two decreasing exponential terms:

$$C(t) = \frac{D}{V_c}\left[\frac{k_{21} - \alpha}{\beta - \alpha} \cdot e^{-\alpha t} + \frac{k_{21} - \beta}{\alpha - \beta} \cdot e^{-\beta t}\right] \qquad (7.8)$$

With (Figure 7.3a):

α: slope of the first linear phase [ln(concentration) vs time] corresponding to the rapid monoexponential decreasing phase (time^{-1}; e.g. h^{-1});

β: slope of the second linear phase [ln(concentration) vs time] corresponding to the slow monoexponential decreasing phase (time^{-1});

k_{12}: rate constant for transfer of drug from central to peripheral compartment (time^{-1});

k_{21}: rate constant for transfer of drug from peripheral to central compartment (time^{-1});

V_c: apparent volume of distribution (ml) of the central (first) compartment. It can be calculated from the administrated dose (total amount) and corresponding concentration, i.e. concentration C_0 associated to the initial time t_0:

$$V_c = \frac{D}{C_0}$$ (7.9)

Equation 7.8 can be simply written under the form:

$$C(t) = A \cdot e^{-\alpha t} + B \cdot e^{-\beta t}$$ (7.10)

With:

$$\alpha + \beta = k_{12} + k_{21} + k_e$$ (7.11)

$$\alpha. \beta = k_{21}.k_e$$ (7.12)

$$A + B = C(0) = C_0$$ (7.13)

The transfer rate constants k_{12}, k_{21} and k_e are also termed microconstants and can be expressed in relation to the macroconstants α, β, A and B (more easy to estimate from the data) (Figure 7.3):

$$k_e = \frac{\alpha \cdot \beta \cdot (A + B)}{A \cdot \beta + \beta \cdot \alpha}$$ (7.14)

$$k_{12} = \frac{A \cdot B \cdot (\beta - \alpha)^2}{(A + B)(A \cdot \beta - B \cdot \alpha)}$$ (7.15)

$$k_{21} = \frac{A \cdot \beta + B \cdot \alpha}{A + B}$$ (7.16)

From the semi-logarithmic plot, extrapolation of the terminal linear phase to the ordinate axis (ln(concentration)) gives the intercept which corresponds to the logarithm of the macroconstant B (Figure 7.3a). This extrapolated line has a slope equal to β and represents the biologic processes that are involved in the disposition of drug; the early (rapid) phase represents a distributive phase of drug in tissues. Therefore, subtracting early times' values (x_1', x_2') of the extrapolated line from observed plasma concentrations (x_1, x_2) at the same times in the distributive phase leads to a number of residual values (x_1-x_1', x_2-x_2') that represent all other processes that, with disposition, influence the early sharp decline of plasma concentration (Figure 7.3a). The line joining such residuals has a slope and intercept equal to the macroconstants α and $\ln(A)$, respectively (Ritschel and Kearn, 1999; Bouroujerdi, 2002).

II.3.3. One-Compartment Model with First-Order Input and First-Order Output

First-order input means proportionality between increase in concentration of inside compartment and the total concentration in outside source. In other words, the amount at the source site is gradually absorbed/transferred to the inside compartment through a driving force resulting in a concentration gradient. Such a driving transfer force corresponds to a passive diffusion which results in a first order transfer kinetics. Therefore, the input or absorption rate from the outside source to inside compartment can be defined as :

$$\text{Input rate} = k_a.A_a \qquad (7.17)$$

Where k_a is the absorption rate constant (time^{-1}) and A_a is the absorbable or bioavailable amount of metabolite (or drug) which escapes from degradation and/or elimination at the source site (Bouroujerdi, 2002).

Model with first-order input and output can be illustrated by oral (or *per os*) administration of a drug which will transit the gastrointestinal tract to systemic circulation before to be eliminated into a single phase (Figure 7.2b). This model is also applicable to any metabolite which diffuses from outside source to inside compartment from which the elimination will occur without interruption by additional transfer phase.

The mathematical formulation of the first-order input and output model uses two exponential terms, $-e^{-k_a t}$ and $+e^{-k_e t}$, representing the increasing and decreasing phases, respectively (Figure 7.2b):

$$C(t) = C_0 \cdot (e^{-k_e t} - e^{-k_a t}) = \underbrace{\frac{F \cdot D \cdot k_a}{V \cdot (k_a - k_e)}}_{C_0} (e^{-k_e t} - e^{-k_a t}) \quad (7.18)$$

$$C(t) = \underbrace{\frac{F \cdot D \cdot k_a}{V \cdot (k_a - k_e)} \cdot e^{-k_e t}}_{\text{Elimination}} - \underbrace{\frac{F \cdot D \cdot k_a}{V \cdot (k_a - k_e)} \cdot e^{-k_a t}}_{\text{Absorption}}$$

With:

C_0: hypothetical concentration corresponding to initial concentration that would have been observed in the case where a dose equal to $A_a = F.D$ was instantaneously inputed.

D: orally administrated dose (μg).

V: apparent volume of distribution (ml).

k_a: absorption rate constant (time^{-1}, e.g. h^{-1}).

k_e: elimination rate constant (time^{-1}).

F: fraction ($0 \leq \ \leq 1$) of compound (drug) that reaches the central compartment (e.g. systemic circulation) from the source site (e.g. gastrointestinal system); $F=1$ for a fully absorbed metabolite (drug) (e.g. across the gastrointestinal tract) ($A_a = D$); $F=0$ for completely unabsorbed metabolite (drug).

For orally administrated drug and under the condition of proportionality between dose D and concentration $C(t)$, the bioavailability fraction F can be calculated from the ratio:

$$F = \frac{AUC_{po}}{AUC_{IV}} \cdot \frac{D_{IV}}{D_{po}} \quad (7.19)$$

Where AUC_{po}, AUC_{IV}, D_{po} and D_{IV} are area under curves and administrated doses in the cases of oral way and bolus intravenous injection, respectively.

The apparent volume of distribution V_d can be calculated by the following formula (Eq. 7.20 or 7.21):

$$V_d = \frac{D \cdot F}{C_0} \cdot \left(\frac{k_a}{k_a - k_e} \right) \tag{7.20}$$

$$V_d = \frac{D \cdot F}{k_e \cdot AUC} = \frac{Cl_{tot}}{k_e} \tag{7.21}$$

With:

D: orally administrated dose.

C_0: initial concentration determined graphically from the intercept $\ln(C_0)$ of extrapolated linear phase to the ln(concentration) axis (Figure 7.2b).

AUC: area under the curve of the orally administrated compound.

F: bioavailability fraction.

k_a: absorption rate constant.

k_e: elimination rate constant.

Cl_{tot}: total clearance, i.e. the hypothetical volume of distribution (in ml) of the compound which is cleared per unit of time (ml/min or ml/h) by all the pathway of compound removal (renal, hepatic, and other pathways of elimination).

II.3.4. Two-Compartments Model with First-Order Input and First-Order Output

This model can be applied when the concentration $C(t)$ in central compartment reaches gradually a peak then decreases according to two phases (Figure 7.3b). The kinetic profile of concentrations $C(t)$ is governed by three successive processes consisting of absorption, distribution and elimination (Figure 7.5). This can be mathematically formulated by a sum of three exponential terms, one increasing representing the absorption phase and two decreasing representing distribution and elimination phases:

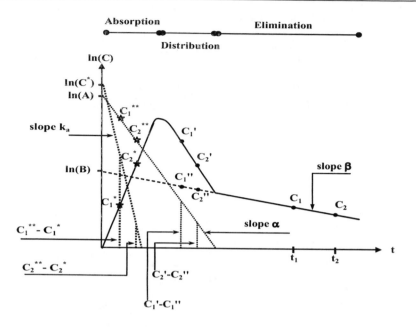

Figure 7.5. Graphical determination of macroconstants β, α, k_a, B, A and C* of first-order input and output compartment model from the slopes and intercepts of three extrapolated lines drawn from observed and residual values extracted from the three kinetic phases (elimination, distribution and absorption).

$$C(t) = \underbrace{B \cdot e^{-\beta t} + A \cdot e^{-\alpha t}}_{\textbf{decreasing phases}} \underbrace{- C^* \cdot e^{-k_a \cdot t}}_{\textbf{Increasing phase}} \qquad (7.22)$$

With:

$$A = \frac{F \cdot D \cdot k_a}{V_c} \cdot \frac{(k_{21} - \alpha)}{(k_a - \alpha) \cdot (\beta - \alpha)} \qquad (7.23)$$

$$B = \frac{F \cdot D \cdot k_a}{V_c} \cdot \frac{(k_{21} - \beta)}{(k_a - \beta) \cdot (\alpha - \beta)} \qquad (7.24)$$

$$C^* = \frac{F \cdot D \cdot k_a}{V_c} \cdot \frac{(k_{21} - k_a)}{(k_a - \alpha) \cdot (\beta - k_a)} \qquad (7.25)$$

With:

F: bioavailability, i.e. fraction ($0 \leq \leq 1$) of compound (drug) that reaches the central compartment (e.g. systemic circulation) from the source site (e.g. gastrointestinal system)

D: orally administrated dose (µg).

V_c: apparent distribution volume of central compartment (ml).

k_a: absorption rate constant (time^{-1}; h^{-1} or min^{-1}).

k_e: elimination rate constant (time^{-1}; h^{-1} or min^{-1}).

k_{12}: Rate constant for transfer of drug from central to peripheral compartment (time^{-1}) (Figure 7.3b).

k_{21}: Rate constant for transfer of drug from peripheral to central compartment (time^{-1}).

The three positive parameters A, B and C^* given by Eqs. 7.23-7.25 correspond to the exponential of intercepts of extrapolated lines having α, β and k_a as slopes (on semi-logarithmic plot) (Figures 7.3b, 7.5) (Ritschel and Kearn, 1999). By considering that $C(0)=0$ and by setting time $t=0$ in Eq. 7.22, the three exponential terms become equal to 1, and the hypothetic initial concentration C^* can be defined as the sum of macroconstants A and B:

$$C^* = A + B \qquad\qquad (7.26)$$

II.3.5. Zero-Order Input Model

Zero-order input can be identified by saturable processes leading to steady state levels. Starting from a continuous secretion or infusion, the concentration of a compound will show a fast increase followed by a braking due to a gradual compensation between input and output (elimination) processes. A balance between input and output can be reached after input duration T superior or equal to five elimination half-life (5 $t_{1/2}$) of the compound (Figure 2.2). In such a case, the concentration will be maintained around a steady state level C_{ss}.

Stopping secretion/supplying of compound before or after C_{ss} level results in immediate elimination phase appearing as abrupt decreasing in concentration curve (Figure 7.6b-d). Such cases will be presented in the next sections concerning models with zero-order input and first-order output (§ II.3.6-II.3.7).

The increase of concentration with time during the infusion process is given by an analytical function in which C_{ss} (the "target" concentration) interacts with an increasing term $(1 - e^{-ke.t})$ comprised between 0 (for t=0) and 1 (for t=+∞):

$$C(t) = \frac{R}{V \cdot k_e}(1 - e^{-k_e \cdot t}) = C_{SS} \cdot (1 - e^{-k_e \cdot t}) \qquad (7.27)$$

with:

R: the infusion rate (μg/h)

V: apparent volume of distribution (ml)

k_e: elimination rate constant (time^{-1})

Equation (7.27) shows that for t=+∞, the exponential term becomes null and $C(t)$ becomes equal to C_{ss}. The infusion model is also applicable to repeated drug administrations at infinitely small time intervals (Ritschel and Kearn, 1999).

Increase in infusion rate R results in increase in steady state level (Figure 7.6a), but the time necessary to reach any SS level remains unchanged and close to 5 $t_{1/2}$ (Figure 7.6a, c; Figure 2.2).

II.3.6. One-Compartment Model with Zero-Order Input and First-Order Output

This model is applied when the kinetics of compound consists of a continuous secretion or infusion phase for a duration T followed by a strict elimination phase starting at t=T, i.e. when the secretion/infusion is stopped (Figure 7.6b-c).

The infusion duration T represents a lag time between the beginning of infusion and that of elimination. It results that concentration C_T cumulated during the infusion duration T represents the initial concentration for the next elimination phase (at t=T). On this basis, the mathematical formulation of elimination phase in this model is analogous to that one-compartment with instantaneous input and first-order output (Eq. 7.3), with the difference that "C_0" is a function of time, noted C_T (Eq. 7.28):

$$C(t) = \overbrace{\underbrace{\frac{R}{V_d \cdot k_e}}_{C_{ss}} \cdot \underbrace{(1 - e^{-k_e T})}_{\text{Infusion}}}^{C_T} \cdot \underbrace{e^{-k_e(t-T)}}_{\text{Elimination}}^{\text{Lag}}$$

(7.28)

With:

R: infusion rate (e.g. µg/h)
V_d: apparent volume of distribution (ml)
k_e: elimination rate constant (e.g. h^{-1})
T: infusion duration (e.g. h^{-1})
t: time from the beginning of infusion (h)
C_{ss} : steady state concentration (e.g. µg/ml)
C_T : Concentration reached at the end of infusion phase (e.g. µg/ml)

Increase in infusion rate R results in increase in C_T and C_{ss} (Figure 7.6a, b). Beyond infusion duration of 5 elimination half-life ($T \geq 5t_{1/2}$), the reached concentration C_T tends to C_{ss} (Figure 7.6c). The parameter k_e can be graphically determined from the elimination phase by the same extrapolation way presented in figure 7.2a.

II.3.7. Two-Compartment Model with Zero-Order Input and First-Order Output

This model is applied for a compound which is secreted/infused for a certain time T then eliminated according to two (fast and slow) phases (Figure 7.6d). Its mathematical formulation implies a sum of two terms, each one combining increasing with decreasing exponential functions:

$$C(t) = \frac{R \cdot (k_{21} - \alpha)(1 - e^{-\alpha T})}{V_c \cdot \alpha \cdot (\alpha - \beta)} \cdot e^{-\alpha t} + \frac{R \cdot (\beta - k_{21})(1 - e^{-\beta T})}{V_c \cdot \beta \cdot (\alpha - \beta)} \cdot e^{-\beta t}$$

(7.29)

$$C(t) = \frac{R}{V_c \cdot (\alpha - \beta)} \cdot \left[\frac{(k_{21} - \alpha)(1 - e^{-\alpha T})}{\alpha} \cdot e^{-\alpha t} + \frac{(\beta - k_{21})(1 - e^{-\beta T})}{\beta} \cdot e^{-\beta t} \right]$$

With:

k_{21}: Rate constant for transfer from the peripheral to the central compartment (h^{-1})

α: Fast disposition rate constant (h^{-1})

β: Slow disposition rate constant (h^{-1})

R: Infusion rate $(\mu g/h)$

V_c: Apparent volume of distribution of the central compartment (ml)

T: Infusion duration, i.e. lag time between start of infusion phase and that of elimination phase (h)

t: Time since start of infusion (h)

The macroconstants α and β are graphically determined from a postinfusion curve by the same way than from a spontaneous input curve (Figure 7.3a).

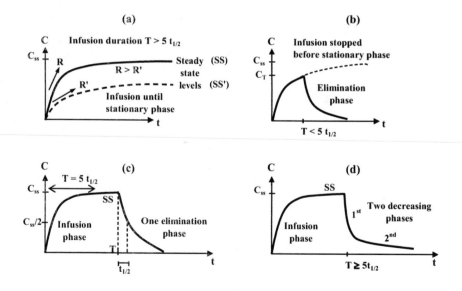

Figure 7.6. Different zero-order input models: (a) no output model; one-compartment model with first-order output starting before (b) and after (c) SS level; (d) two-compartment model with first-order output. (a): R, R' represents two different infusion rates (R>R') leading to two different SS levels (SS >SS').

II.3.8. One-Compartment Model with Michaelis Menten-Type Output

This model is applied when the elimination from the compartment is a saturable process. This can be the case of many biological transports which are enzyme-controlled (Gillespie, 1993; Piotrovskij and Van Peer, 1998; Chappel, 1999; Derendorf and Meibohm, 1999). In this case, the elimination rate k_e (Eq. 7.1) is not proportional to $C(t)$ but depends on $C(t)$; consequently, the rate of decline of concentration dC/dt could obey Michaelis-Menten kinetics:

$$\frac{dC(t)}{dt} = -\frac{V_{max}}{K_m + C(t)} \cdot C(t) \tag{7.30}$$

Where:

V_{max} is the limit or maximal velocity of the process (elimination)

K_m is the Michaelis Menten constant, i.e. the concentration remaining to be eliminated if the rate has decreased to 50% of V_{max}. In other words, it is the concentration that produces 50% of the maximal velocity V_{max} ($K_m \rightarrow v=0.5V_{max}$).

Under saturable elimination processes, Michaelis-Menten kinetics can be graphically identified by a less concave decay of $C(t)$ compared to the exponential decay (Figure 7.7a). In semi-logarithmic plot, the ratio V_{max}/K_m can be estimated from the terminal slope (Figure 7.7b) (Holz and Fahr, 2001).

Compared to Eq. 7.1, Eq. 7.30 shows that the proportionality is not constant but a function of $C(t)$. In place of k_e, the proportionality term is represented by $V_{max}/(K_m + C(t))$ which depends on $C(t)$. Eq. 7.30 cannot be integrated analytically so that $C(t)$ must be computed numerically.

In enzyme kinetics, Eq. 7.30 is used to fit the reaction velocity or metabolism rate v which is experimentally measured in relation to substrate (drug) concentration C:

$$v = \frac{V_{max} \cdot C}{K_m + C} \tag{7.31}$$

By knowing the substrate (drug) concentrations C and corresponding reaction velocities v, the Eq. 7.31 can be linearized by inverse transformation from which the coefficients V_{max} and K_m can be graphically determined (Figure 7.8) (Bonate, 2006):

$$\frac{1}{v} = \frac{K_m + C}{V_{max} \cdot C} = \frac{K_m}{V_{max}} \cdot \frac{1}{C} + \frac{1}{V_{max}}$$ (7.32)

The Eq. 7.31 represents a linear model according to the variable $(1/C)$. Its unknown parameters V_{max} and K_m can be graphically determined from the slope (K_m/V_{max}) and the intercept $(1/V_{max})$ of the plot $1/v$ vs $1/C$ (Figure 7.8), the equation of which can be determined by using standard linear regression (Zar, 1999).

Michaelis-Menten model is also used in pharmacology to fit the transfer of drug effect E from systemic circulation to "effect compartment" (Derendorf and Meibohm, 1999; Hu et al., 1995; Jacobs and Williams, 1993):

$$E(t) = \frac{E_{max} \cdot C(t)}{IC_{50} + C(t)}$$ (7.33)

Where:

$E(t)$ is the drug effect at time t, E_{max} is the maximal effect and IC_{50} is the concentration that produces 50% of E_{max}.

Eqs. 7.31 and 7.33 are applied for one-site enzyme model, i.e. when the interaction between substrate (drug) and enzyme occurs at only one receptor site. However, by considering the multimeric receptor case, the cooperativity degree of an enzyme can be expressed by means of the Hill equation (Hill, 1910):

$$v = \frac{V_{max} \cdot C^h}{K_{0.5}{}^h + C^h}$$ (7.34)

In Eq. 7.34, the parameter V_{max} plays the same role than the maximal velocity of Michaelis-Menten equation (Eq. 7.31). $K_{0.5}$ (analogous to K_m of Eq. 7.31) defines the concentration of substrate at which $v=0.5V_{max}$. The parameter h, called Hill's parameter, is used as cooperativity index between the enzyme and the substrate: cooperativity is a phenomenon observed when a multimeric receptor (enzyme) attaches a same ligand at several non-independent fixation sites. The occupation of the first site(s) by the ligand results in a structural modification which will have repercussions on the properties of remaining free sites. The cooperativity occurs when the occupation of the first sites increases the affinity of the remaining sites for the next ligand molecules: "the first fixed ligands help the following ones to be installed". A higher Hill's parameter h indicates a higher cooperativity degree. Non-cooperative enzyme corresponds to the Michaelis-Menten model where $h=1$. Therefore, cooperativity (or positive cooperativity) means $h>1$. When inverse phenomenon occurs it is called anti-cooperativity (or negative cooperativity) with $h<1$.

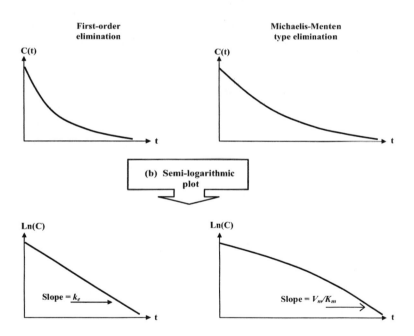

Figure 7.7. Comparison between first-order and Michaelis-Menten type eliminations based on concentration-time (a) and semi-logarihtmic (b) plots. From concentration-time plot (a), Michaelis-Menten type elimination is less concave than exponential elimination. From semi-logarithmic plot (b), exponential elimination shows a well lined plot after semilogarithmic transformation.

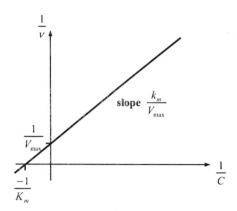

Figure 7.8. Graphical determination of Michaelis-Menten parameters from the reciprocal of reaction velocity (metabolism rate) versus the reciprocal of substrate (drug) concentration.

III. STOCHASTIC MODELING OF KINETICS OF METABOLIC SYSTEMS

III.1. GENERAL CONCEPTS

The term stochastic is applied to random processes evolving generally in time with probabilities varying according to some laws. The modeling of such random variation laws represents a fundamental question which can be solved by using appropriate probability density functions (pdf). The resulting models, called stochastic or probabilistic models, give at any time of the variation field the occurrence probability of a random variable characterizing the studied process. This, by opposition to the deterministic models giving well determined values characterizing the system states. Beyond a single random variable, stochastic process can be studied on the basis of a family of random variables varying in time.

Stochastic models differ also from deterministic ones by the notion of elementary component on the basis of which models will be established:

In stochastic modeling, the elementary component is the particle (e.g. metabolite molecule) the random behavior(s) of which will be formalized by using random variables associated to random laws (Purdue, 1979; Gardiner, 2004). However, the deterministic approaches start from small variations which will be expressed in terms of differential equations leading to analytical or numerical functions. In summary, the deterministic models are built on the basis of mass concept versus particle concept and elementary events in stochastic modeling.

Basically, a stochastic process can be illustrated by the classic example of Brownian movement or random walk: Brownian movement consists of the free movement of a molecule considered independently from the other identical molecules. Such a movement is sensitively rectilinear and uniform taking steps of equal size in any direction (Figure 7.9a). Moreover, the different random walk steps tend to cancel each other out.

There are two important questions concerning such a stochastic process:

1) What is the distribution of random walkers as function of time?
2) What is the average distance that a single walker is expected to go in a given time?

For 1), the spatial distribution of random walkers is well described by a Gaussian or normal distribution (Figure 7.9b). The total walk as well as each step have Gaussian probability distributions. In these cases, the whole is similar to each of the parts, and in this sense, a Gaussian random walk is self-similar. Likewise, a purposeful walk is self-similar: each step looks like a miniature copy of the whole walk.

For 2), although, the walkers are assumed to have uniform and rectilinear movements, their path take so many twists and turns that the total displacement (from the start to the end of their walks) is, on average, proportional to the square root of past time ($\sqrt{t}$) (Figure 7.9a). For purposeful movement condensing all the random walk steps in a single direction, the start-to-end displacement increases at a rate proportional to t (Figure 7.9c). This shows the existence of orders in the apparent disorder resulting from the random walk of particle.

These two questions concerning the random walk process can be asked in terms of any other random processes and variables.

III.2. General Methodological Tools

To analyse stochastically a system (e.g. metabolic system), all the particles (metabolite molecules) are assumed to be identical and independent along the considered time range (Purdue, 1979). Then, elementary events generating the studied functional system will be statistically modeled by appropriate pdf fitting the behavior frequencies of random variables from the observed experimental data. Random variables are diversified and depends on the studied functional aspects of system. For instance, by reference to stochastic compartment models, random variables can consist of (Matis and Wehrly, 1990; Wimmer et al., 1999; Lansky, 1996):

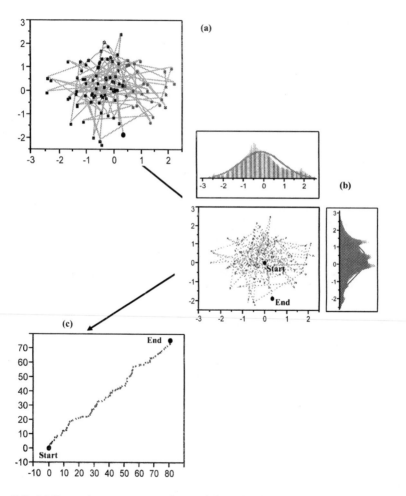

Figure 7.9. (a) Brownian movement of a particle consisting of its random walk in infinity of possible directions from start to end; 100 steps are shown. (b) The set of all the step lengths of the random walk follow a Gaussian distribution. (c) A purposeful walker starts from the coordinate (0,0) and takes steps in a single direction; the distance due to all the accumulated steps between start and end is proportional to the past time t since start.

- The single visit or transit time S_{ij} of a particle coming from compartment i to compartment j.
- The transit time R_{ij} during a single visit in compartment i of a particle whose next transfer will be to compartment j.
- The residence time in the system of a particle originating from compartment i.
- The residence time that a particle originating from compartment i accumulates in compartment j during all its visits $i \rightarrow j$. This can be conceived as the sum of N_{ij} transit times S_{ij} of the particle during N_{ij} single visits from compartment i to compartment j.
- The number of visits N_{ij} in compartment j of a particle originating from compartment i.
- The cycle time Tk, i.e. time that particle takes to perform a whole system circulation to return to a same point.
- The number of system cycles that a particle performs before its elimination.

By considering the shape of experimental data curve, an appropriate pdf can be used to fit the the the whole process responsible for the observed data. The pdfs are advantageously flexible show a flexibility advantage to curve fitting because they combine few parameters to generate different shapes. These parameters can be classified in two types consisting of scale and shape parameters. Among the pdfs, binomial, Poisson and geometric laws can be applied to discrete random variables as success numbers (e.g. number of visits, number of cycles, etc.). Normal, logistic, Weibull and gamma laws can be used to continuous random variables as residence, transit or cycle times of particle.

From the appropriate pdf $p(t)$ depicting a considered random process, the kinetic variations of the final governed variable $X(t)$ (e.g. concentration) can be stochastically estimated from the product of $p(t)$ by the whole quantity X_{wh} of such a variable in the system:

$$X(t) = X_{wh} \times p(t) = p(t) \cdot \int_{0}^{\infty} X(t) dt \qquad (7.35)$$

$$\Leftrightarrow \qquad p(t) = \frac{X(t)}{\int_{0}^{\infty} X(t) dt} \qquad (7.36)$$

The probability given by Eq. 7.36 assumes that all the actor particles are identical, behave independently of one to another, and once eliminated they never return into the system (Wimmer et al., 1999).

By reference (by analogy) to the random walk model, the toal quantity X_{wh} integrates all the "random walkers" which start out from the same place at the same time. As time proceeds, such a high concentration of random walkers spreads out, invading regions or phases of lower concentrations. Such a distribution of "random walkers" concentration will be conditioned by the stochastic process represented by the corresponding pdf. Thus, the fitting of the kinetic variations of metabolite concentration $C(t)$ can be fitted on the basis of the product:

$$C(t) = p(t) \cdot \int_0^\infty C(t)dt = p(t) \cdot AUC(0,\infty) \qquad (7.37)$$

Where:

$AUC(0,\infty)$ is the area under the concentration-time curve.
$p(t)$ is the probability calculated from the appropriate pdf.

In the next sections, stochastic modeling of different concentration-time curves will be illustrated on the basis of generalized Weibull distribution which represents one among the most flexible pdfs.

III.3. Stochastic Fitting of concentration-Time Curves Based on Generalized Weibull Distribution

The generalized Weibull distribution (GWD) provides a high flexibility through its four scale and shape parameters. The variations of these parameters result in contraction or stretching in the pdf curve leading to fit different kinetic models. For $t>0$, the pdf $p(t)$ of GWD is defined by (Heikkilä, 1999):

$$p(t) = \frac{\log\theta}{2^\lambda - 1} \cdot \frac{\lambda\gamma}{\beta} \left(\frac{t}{\beta}\right)^{\gamma-1} \left[\left(\frac{t}{\beta}\right)^\gamma + 1\right]^{\lambda-1} e^{-\left\{\left(\frac{\log\theta}{2^\lambda-1}\right)\left[\left(\left(\frac{t}{\beta}\right)^\gamma+1\right)^\lambda-1\right]\right\}}$$

$$(7.38)$$

Where:

t represents the random variable; time in this case (e.g. residence time of particle).

β (scale parameter) defines the unit of measurement of the time scale.

γ controls the initial level of ordinate axis; it is equal to 1 when the curve has a finite initial value and it varies between 0 and 1 ($0 < \gamma < 1$) when the curve is unbounded at $t=0$ (Figure 7.10d).

λ (shape parameter) induces a non linear contraction or stretching of the time scale for $\lambda < 1$ and $\lambda > 1$, respectively.

θ (shape parameter) plays a role in the general form of the curve. For example, for $\lambda=1$ and $\theta=e$, the GWD reduces to the ordinary Weibull distribution (Eq. 7.39) (Hoyland and Rausand, 1994):

$$p(t) = \frac{\gamma}{\beta} \cdot \left(\frac{t}{\beta}\right)^{\gamma-1} e^{-\left(\frac{t}{\beta}\right)^{\gamma}} \qquad (7.39)$$

The GWD pdf (Eq. 7.38) can be reparametrized to fit different kinetic models such as (Heikkilä, 1999):

- Instantaneous input with first order output;
- First order input and output.

The fittings of these models will be illustrated in the following sections.

Kinetic models of concentration are developed by multiplying the pdf $p(t)$ by a positive parameter ω which integrate the basic conditions of the considered model. The parameter ω plays a similar role than AUC($0, \infty$) in Eq. 7.37.

$$C(t) = \omega. \, p(t) \qquad\qquad (\omega > 0) \qquad\qquad (7.40)$$

In stochastic fitting, the number of compartment is not required because the shape and scale of model curvature are directly controlled through variations of the pdf parameters.

III.3.1. Generalized Weibull Distribution Applied to Instantaneous Input with First Order Output Kinetic Model

Under instantaneous input and first order output conditions, the concentration-time curve decreases monotonously from initial level $C(0)$ representing the initial and whole concentration administrated in the system (Chapter 7, § II.3.1).

The monotonous decreasing curve can be fitted by means of a GWD by parametrizing ω (Eq. 7.40) under the form (Heikkilä, 1999):

$$\omega = \frac{\alpha\beta(2^{\lambda}-1)}{\log(\theta)\lambda\gamma} \tag{7.41}$$

When this parameterization is associated with the value of $\gamma=1$, it attributes to the model a finite initial value α corresponding to the concentration $C(0)$ (Eqs 7.42-7.45) (Figure 7.10a). More precisely, $\alpha=C(0)$ corresponds to $\lim_{t\to0+} C(t)$ (with $\gamma=1$). However, for $0<\gamma\leq1$, the curve is unbounded at initial time $t=0$ (Figure 7.10d).

By combining Eqs. 7.40 and 7.41, the general equation of $C(t)$ can be determined for $t>0$ by:

$$C(t) = \omega \times p(t) = \frac{\alpha\beta(2^{\lambda}-1)}{\log(\theta)\lambda\gamma} \times \frac{\log\theta}{2^{\lambda}-1} \cdot \frac{\lambda\gamma}{\beta}\left(\frac{t}{\beta}\right)^{\gamma-1}\left[\left(\frac{t}{\beta}\right)^{\gamma}+1\right]^{\lambda-1} e^{-\left\{\left(\frac{\log\theta}{2^{\lambda}-1}\right)\left[\left(\left(\frac{t}{\beta}\right)^{\gamma}+1\right)^{\lambda}-1\right]\right\}}$$

$$C(t) = \alpha \cdot \left(\frac{t}{\beta}\right)^{\gamma-1}\left[\left(\frac{t}{\beta}\right)^{\gamma}+1\right]^{\lambda-1} e^{-\left\{\left(\frac{\log\theta}{2^{\lambda}-1}\right)\left[\left(\left(\frac{t}{\beta}\right)^{\gamma}+1\right)^{\lambda}-1\right]\right\}} \tag{7.42}$$

This model has six parameters, α, β, γ, δ, λ, θ. By setting $\lambda=\delta/\gamma$ and by introducing the restriction $\theta=2^{\lambda}$, the concentration-time model can be brought down to four dimension parameter space:

$$C(t) = \alpha \cdot \left(\frac{t}{\beta}\right)^{\gamma-1}\left[\left(\frac{t}{\beta}\right)^{\gamma}+1\right]^{\frac{\delta}{\gamma}-1} \cdot \exp\left(-\left\{\left(\frac{\log\left[2^{\left(\frac{\delta}{\gamma}\right)}\right]}{2^{\left(\frac{\delta}{\gamma}\right)}-1}\right)\left[\left(\left(\frac{t}{\beta}\right)^{\gamma}+1\right)^{\frac{\delta}{\gamma}}-1\right]\right\}\right) \tag{7.43}$$

In this equation, the parameters δ and γ in the exponents are proper shape parameters (Figure 7.10c, d). The parameter α and β determines the concentration and time scales, respectively (Figure 7.10a, b); they are shape invariant (Heikkilä, 1999).

Finally, by considering the condition $\gamma=1$ satisfying a finite initial concentration $\alpha=C(0)$, the model can be simplified to be (Figure 7.10a-c):

$$C(t) = \alpha \cdot \left[\left(\frac{t}{\beta}\right)+1\right]^{\delta-1} \exp\left(-\left\{\left(\frac{\log(2^\delta)}{2^\delta-1}\right)\left[\left(\left(\frac{t}{\beta}\right)+1\right)^\delta -1\right]\right\}\right) \quad (7.44)$$

One can check that α corresponds to the initial concentration $C(0)$ by setting $t=0$ in Eq. 7.44. This equation reduces to the ordinary one-exponential model when $\gamma=1$ and $\delta=1$:

$$C(t) = \alpha \cdot e^{-\log(2)\frac{t}{\beta}} \quad (7.45)$$

The model (7.44) corresponding to $\gamma=1$, goes through the point $(\beta, \alpha/2)$ which is equal to $(t_{1/2}, C(0)/2)$ (Figure 7.10c). The forth parameter δ can be indirectly determined from θ which can be estimated from the AUC$(0,\infty)$ and AUC$(0,\beta)$ calculated by the trapezoid rule (Eq. 7.6):

$$AUC(0,\infty) = \int_0^\infty C(t)dt = \omega$$
$$AUC(0,\beta) = \int_0^\beta C(t)dt = \omega - \frac{\omega}{\theta} \qquad \Rightarrow \theta = \frac{\omega}{\omega - AUC(0,\beta)} \quad (7.46)$$

Therefore, the parameter δ can be calculated from:

$$\theta = 2^\lambda = 2^{\delta/\gamma} = 2^{\delta/1} = 2^\delta \quad \Leftrightarrow \quad \delta = \log_2(\theta) \quad (7.47)$$

This calculation procedure is not optimal statistical method for determining estimates of the parameters. However, it can be used to obtain estimates that can be helpfully used as initial values to solve the system by a non linear optimization program (Seber and Wild, 1989; Bonate, 2006).

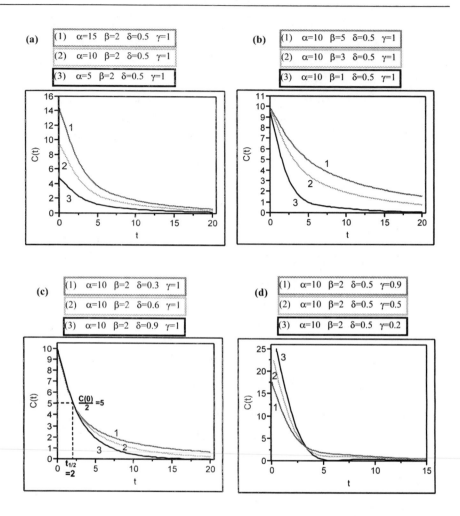

Figure 7.10. Variations, one at once, of shape and scale parameters in the equation 7.43 based on Weibull distribution leading to fit different monotonously decreasing kinetic curves $C(t)$.

III.3.2. Generalized Weibull Distribution Applied to First Order Input and Output Kinetic Model

The GWD can be reparametrized under some constraints to fit a first-order input and output model, with a kinetic curve consisting of a null initial value followed by a peak then a final decreasing phase (Figure 7.5). Such a general curve shape can be obtained for $\gamma > 1$ (Figure 7.11) (Heikkilä, 1999). To fit such a one-peak curve, the shape-invariant parameters α and β have to correspond to C_{max} and t_{max}, respectively (Figure 7.1b). The requirement $\beta=t_{max}$ is ensured by the following restriction on the general shape parameter θ:

$$\log \theta = \frac{(\gamma + \gamma\lambda - 2) \cdot (2^{\lambda} - 1)}{2^{\lambda} \gamma\lambda} \tag{7.48}$$

Moreover, the reparameterization of the AUC-like (ω) of Eq. 7.41 ensures that $\alpha=C_{max}$:

$$\omega = \frac{2\alpha\beta\theta}{\gamma + \gamma\lambda - 2} \tag{7.49}$$

From these basic considerations and parameterizations, the kinetic model $C(t)$ can be obtained from the product $\omega.p(t)$ (Eq. 7.40) leading to the following equation:

$$C(t) = \alpha \left(\frac{t}{\beta}\right)^{\gamma-1} \left[\frac{1}{2}\left(\frac{t}{\beta}\right)^{\gamma} + \frac{1}{2}\right]^{\frac{\gamma+\gamma\lambda}{\gamma}-2} \exp\left\{-\frac{\gamma+\gamma\lambda-2}{\gamma+\gamma\lambda-\gamma}\left\{\left[\frac{1}{2}\left(\frac{t}{\beta}\right)^{\gamma} + \frac{1}{2}\right]^{\frac{\gamma+\gamma\lambda}{\gamma}-1} - 1\right\}\right\} \tag{7.50}$$

By introducing the reparametrization $\kappa=\gamma+\gamma\lambda$, the equation (7.50) can be simplified to:

$$C(t) = \alpha \left(\frac{t}{\beta}\right)^{\gamma-1} \left[\frac{1}{2}\left(\frac{t}{\beta}\right)^{\gamma} + \frac{1}{2}\right]^{\frac{\kappa}{\gamma}-2} \exp\left\{-\frac{\kappa-2}{\kappa-\gamma}\left\{\left[\frac{1}{2}\left(\frac{t}{\beta}\right)^{\gamma} + \frac{1}{2}\right]^{\frac{\kappa}{\gamma}-1} - 1\right\}\right\} \tag{7.51}$$

This model has four parameters: β and α are invariant shape parameters corresponding to t_{max} and C_{max}, respectively. All the curves issued from Eq. 7.51 go through the point (β, α) corresponding to (t_{max}, C_{max}) (Figure 7.11). The parameters γ (>1) and κ (> max(2,γ)) are shape parameters. A larger value of γ corresponds to a more peaked curve around C_{max} (Figure 7.11). In statistical terms, γ play a role of kurtosis for the curve. The parameter κ primarily regulates the rate of decay in the decreasing part of the curve (Figure

7.11). It can be empirically estimated from the geometric characteristics of the concentration-time curve:

$$\kappa = \frac{2C_{max} \cdot t_{max}}{AUC(0,\infty) - AUC(0,t_{max})} + 2 \qquad (7.52)$$

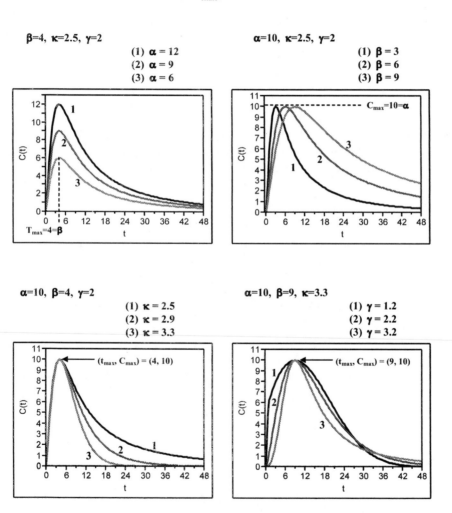

Figure 7.11. Variations, one at once, of shape and scale parameters in the equation 7.51 based on Weibull distribution leading to fit different one-peak kinetic curves C(t).

IV. DYNAMIC STABILITY ANALYSIS
OF METABOLIC SYSTEMS

IV.1. General Background

Biological (metabolic) systems can be analysed on the basis of their ability to opposite or to be subjected to perturbations. This concept is at the basis of a dynamic approach known under the term of stability analysis (Steuer, 2007; Fall et al., 2005):

Stability analysis aims to examine the behavior of a dynamic system around its equilibrium state which can be represented by a stationary regimen (Figure 1.11a). Therefore, the question of stability can be asked in different manners:

- If the system is deviated from the equilibrium, does it return to this state?
- Does small perturbation, moving away the system from its stationary regimen, result in amplifications in time?

Such questions imply the analysis of all the possible perturbations of the system in relation to small variations of its p parameters x_j (e.g. p metabolites' concentrations) in time and the ones with respect to the others (Figure 7.12a).

IV.2. Methodology Based on Jacobian Matrix

The different parameters (variables) x_j of system (e.g. concentrations of different metabolites j) can be linked the ones the others by different time-dependent functions. In other words, the variation of a given parameter in time can depend on other parameters varying in time (e.g. $x_1(t) = x_1 t + 5x_3^2 t$; $x_3(t) = -4x_2 t$). A small perturbation of the system can be mathematically expressed by all the derivatives f_j of such parameters with respect to time:

$$f_j = \frac{dx_j}{dt} \tag{7.53}$$

At equilibrium point, the derivatives of all the parameters x_j with respect to time are null: $f_j = \dfrac{dx_j}{dt} = 0$. Therefore, the equilibrium point of system, $X^*(x_1^*, x_2^*, \ldots, x_p^*)$, can be determined by putting to zero all the derivative functions f_j leading to determine the equilibrium values x_j^* variables x_j. With p parameters x_j ($j=1$ to p), one expects p values x_j^* to calculate from p derivative equations $f_j=0$.

The relative variation of the perturbed system with respect to all its variables x_j can be expressed by the partial derivatives $\dfrac{df_j}{dx_j}$ of all the multivariate flow functions f_j resulting in a ($p \times p$)-dimension matrix J called Jacobian matrix (Figure 7.12a3). The analytical elements of J can be obtained from perturbed time-courses using linear least-squares fitting (Soribas et al., 1998; Diaz-Sierra et al., 1999; Crampin et al., 2004). This method is based on the fact that transients yield responses to small perturbations under steady-state conditions. The mathematical basis for this is that the linear representation constitutes the first-order term of a Taylor series expansion, which is sufficiently accurate in this situation.

The calculus of partial derivatives df_j/dx_j at the equilibrium point $X^*(x_1^*, x_2^*, \ldots, x_p^*)$ gives the Jacobian matrix J^* with ($p \times p$) values. For a metabolic system, J^* describes its dynamical characteristics near the steady state. Analysis of the properties of J^* helps to analyse the stability of the system around the equilibrium point X^*. Such a stability analysis consists in:

- Calculating the eigenvalues λ_j of J^* (there are as much eigenvalues as parameters) (Figure 7.12a4).
- Interpreting their types and signs in terms of stability or non-stability of the system (Figure 7.12a5, 7.12b).

Eigenvalues of a biological (metabolic) system can be real or complex on the hand, and positive or negative on the other hand (Figure 7.12b):

Complex eigenvalues indicate an oscillatory system (Figure 7.12b: II, IV). Inversely, a system with only real eigenvalues is non-oscillatory (Figure 7.12b: I, III, V). The sign of eigenvalue provides information on the convergence or divergence of the system, i.e. on its return or no to stability, respectively: a negative real eigenvalue (negative real part) indicates a stable system, i.e. a system which converges (returns) to steady state (equilibrium) (after disruption) (Figure 7.12b: I, II). A positive real eigenvalue (positive real part) indicates a system which never converges to steady state (Figure 7.12b: IV, V). When some eigenvalues are positive and others are negative, the system has a saddle point, which represents a fragile equilibrium state leading the system to be unstable (Figure 7.12b: III).

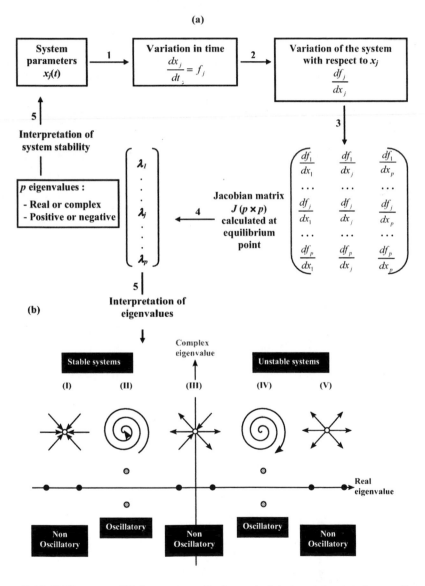

Figure 7.12. Different equilibrium states of a dynamical system interpreted according to the types and signs of the eigenvalues calculated from the Jacobian matrix.

IV.3. Numerical Example of Stability Analysis

Let's consider a hypothetical system with three parameters $x_1(t)$, $x_2(t)$ and $x_3(t)$. The analytical functions of these three time-dependent variables are:

$$x_1(t) = -x_1^2 t + 10 x_2 t = (-x_1^2 + 10 x_2)t$$
$$x_2(t) = -5x_2 t + 3x_3^2 t = (-5x_2 + 3x_3^2)t$$
$$x_3(t) = -5x_1 t - 2x_2^3 t + x_3 t = (-5x_1 - 2x_2^3 + x_3)t$$

The variations of the three concentrations in a small time range are given by the three derivatives functions $f_j(x)$ (Eqs 7.54):

$$f_1(x) = \frac{dx_1}{dt} = -x_1^2 + 10x_2$$

$$f_2(x) = \frac{dx_2}{dt} = -5x_2 + 3x_3^2 \qquad (7.54)$$

$$f_3(x) = \frac{dx_3}{dt} = -5x_1 + 2x_2^3 + x_3$$

The variations of these three flow functions f_j with respect to the parameters x_j are given by the Jacobian matrix J containing the nine ($p \times p$) partial derivatives $\dfrac{df_j(x)}{dx_j}$:

$$J = \begin{pmatrix} \dfrac{df_1(x)}{dx_1} & \dfrac{df_1(x)}{dx_2} & \dfrac{df_1(x)}{dx_3} \\[2mm] \dfrac{df_2(x)}{dx_1} & \dfrac{df_2(x)}{dx_2} & \dfrac{df_2(x)}{dx_3} \\[2mm] \dfrac{df_3(x)}{dx_1} & \dfrac{df_3(x)}{dx_2} & \dfrac{df_3(x)}{dx_3} \end{pmatrix} = \begin{pmatrix} \dfrac{d(-x_1^2+10x_2)}{dx_1} & \dfrac{d(-x_1^2+10x_2)}{dx_2} & \dfrac{d(-x_1^2+10x_2)}{dx_3} \\[2mm] \dfrac{d(-5x_2+3x_3^2)}{dx_1} & \dfrac{d(-5x_2+3x_3^2)}{dx_2} & \dfrac{d(-5x_2+3x_3^2)}{dx_3} \\[2mm] \dfrac{d(-5x_1+2x_2^3+x_3)}{dx_1} & \dfrac{d(-5x_1+2x_2^3+x_3)}{dx_2} & \dfrac{d(-5x_1+2x_2^3+x_3)}{dx_3} \end{pmatrix}$$

The derivations give:

$$J = \begin{pmatrix} -2x_1 & +10 & 0 \\ 0 & -5 & 6x_3 \\ -5 & 6x_2^{\,2} & 1 \end{pmatrix}$$

Now that we know the elements of J, we can fully describe the stability of the system. The point $X^*(x_1^*, x_2^*, x_3^*)=(0, 0, 0)$ represents an equilibrium point at which all the derivatives df_j/dt are null (Eqs. 7.54). At this equilibrium point, the Jacobian matrix J^* is:

$$J^* = \begin{pmatrix} 0 & 10 & 0 \\ 0 & -5 & 0 \\ -5 & 0 & 1 \end{pmatrix}$$

The eigenvalues λ and their associated eigenvectors U of J^* can be determined according to the matricial equation:

$$J^*.U=\lambda.U \Leftrightarrow J^*.U-\lambda.U=0$$
$$\Leftrightarrow (J^*-\lambda.I).U=0 \Leftrightarrow J^*-\lambda.I=0 \tag{7.55}$$

Where I is the identity matrix $(p{\times}p)$. To solve this matricial equation, we should to calculate its determinant; then by putting the determinant to zero, the eigenvalues λ can be determined as solutions of the system. The equation $J^*-\lambda.I=0$ can be written:

$$\begin{pmatrix} 0 & 10 & 0 \\ 0 & -5 & 0 \\ -5 & 0 & 1 \end{pmatrix} - \lambda \begin{pmatrix} 1 & 0 & 0 \\ 0 & 1 & 0 \\ 0 & 0 & 1 \end{pmatrix} = 0$$

$$\Leftrightarrow$$

$$\begin{pmatrix} 0 & 10 & 0 \\ 0 & -5 & 0 \\ -5 & 0 & 1 \end{pmatrix} - \begin{pmatrix} \lambda & 0 & 0 \\ 0 & \lambda & 0 \\ 0 & 0 & \lambda \end{pmatrix} = 0$$

$$\Leftrightarrow$$

$$\begin{pmatrix} -\lambda & 10 & 0 \\ 0 & -5-\lambda & 0 \\ -5 & 0 & 1-\lambda \end{pmatrix} = 0$$

The determinant of this matrix can be written:

$$\det = -\lambda \times \begin{vmatrix} -5-\lambda & 0 \\ 0 & 1-\lambda \end{vmatrix} - 0 \times \begin{vmatrix} 10 & 0 \\ 0 & 1-\lambda \end{vmatrix} - 5 \times \begin{vmatrix} 10 & 0 \\ -5-\lambda & 0 \end{vmatrix}$$

$$= -\lambda \times (-5-\lambda)(1-\lambda) - 0 \times (10 \times (1-\lambda)) - 5 \times (10 \times 0 - (5-\lambda) \times 0)$$

$$= -\lambda \times (-5-\lambda+5\lambda+\lambda^2) = -\lambda(\lambda^2+4\lambda-5)$$

By putting the determinant to zero, a first solution $\lambda_1=0$ can be directly extracted. The two others can be determined by calculating the discriminant Δ of $\lambda^2+4\lambda-5$. One obtains $\Delta = 4^2 + 4 \times 5 = 16 + 20 = 36$. Therefore, the solutions λ_2 and λ_3 can be calculated by:

$$\lambda_2 = \frac{-4+\sqrt{36}}{2} = 1 \qquad \text{and} \qquad \lambda_3 = \frac{-4-\sqrt{36}}{2} = -5$$

The triplet of solutions $(\lambda_1, \lambda_2, \lambda_3)=(0, 1, -5)$ show that there are only real λ values (i.e. non complex values because Δ was not negative). This can be interpreted as a non-oscillatory dynamic system.

Tacking into account the signs of the eigenvalues, both positive and negative values are obtained. This corresponds to a saddle point meaning a fragile equilibrium of the dynamic system: the fact that one eigenvalue is negative and the other positive means that the dynamic system is subjected to both stability attracting and repelling processes. Because they both attract and repel, saddle points provide a stretching and folding that often produces chaos. Saddle points have a special importance in non-linear dynamics. In high dimensional systems, they are the most common type of equilibrium (Sprott, 2003).

REFERENCES

Abraham, R, & Shaw, C. (1981). *Dynamics: The Geometry of Behavior*. The Visual Math. Libr., Aerial Press.

Anderson, D.H., McWilliams, J.G. & Roller T. (1988). The unilateral circulation compartmental model, *Math. Biosci. 89*, 183-208.

Andrews, D. F. (1972). Plots of high-dimensional data. *Biometrics, 28*, 125-136.

Antoniewicz, M.R., Stephanopoulos, G. & Kelleher, J.K. (2006). Evaluation of regression models in metabolic physiology: predicting fluxes from isotopic data without knowledge of the pathway. *Metabolomics, 2*, 41-52.

Arabie, P., De Soete, G., Arabie, P., Hubert, L. J., Hubert, L. J. & De Soete, G. (Eds.) (1996). *Clustering and Classification*. World Scientific Pub. Co. Inc., River Edge, New Jersey.

Aronsson, G., Kellog, R.B. (1978). On a differential equation arising from compartment analysis. *Math. Biosci.*, *38*, 113-122.

Atkinson, D. E. (1977). *Cellular Energy Metabolism and its Regulation*. Academic Press, New York.

Bailey, J.E. (1998). Mathematical modeling and analysis in biochemical engineering: past accomplishments and future opportunities. *Biotechnol. Progr.*, *14*, 8-20.

Barnett V. (1976). The ordering of multivariate data (with discussion). *J. R. Stat. Soc. A, 139*, 318-354.

Barnett, V. (1976). The ordering of multivariate data (with discussion). *J R Stat Soc A, 139*, 318-354.

Barnett, V. & Lewis, T. (1994). *Outliers in statistical data*. Wiley, New York.

Baths, V., Rohit Kumar, V.V., Praneeth G.V.R. & Roy, U. (2009). Graph theoretic approach on metabolomic networks of mycobacteral strains for potential drug targets. *Research Journal of Microbiology*, *4*, 132-137.

Beal, S.L. (1987). Some clarifications regarding moments of residence times with pharmacokinetic models. *J. Pharmacokint. Biopharm.*, *15*, 75-92.

Beard, D.A., Liang, S.D., Qian, H. (2002). Energy balance for analysis of complex metabolic networks. *Biophys. J.*, *83*,79–86.

Blackwood, C. B., Marsh, T., Kim, S. H. & Paul, E. A. (2003). Terminal restriction fragment length polymorphism data analysis for quantitative comparison of microbial communities. *Appl. Environ. Microbiol, 69*, 926-932.

Bonate, P.L. (2006). *Pharmacokinetic-Pharmacodynamic Modeling and Simulation*. Springer, San Antonio, *387*.

Bonarius, H.P.J., Hatzimanikatis, V., Meesters, K.P.H., de Gooijer, C.D., Schmid, G. & Tramper, J. (1996). Metabolomic flux analysis of hybrodoma cells in different culture media using mass balances. *Biotechnol. Bioeng.*, *50*, 299-318.

Boroujerdi, M. (2002). *Pharmacokinetics: Principles and Applications*. McGraw-Hill, New york, *420*.

Box, G. E. P. & Cox, D. R. (1964). An analysis of transformations. *J. R. Stat. Soc. B*, *26*, 211-252.

Box, G. E. P, Hunter, W. G. & Hunter, J. S. (1978). Statistics for Experimenters: an Introduction to Design, Data Analysis and Model Building. Willey, New York.

Brown, G.C., Lakin-Thomas, P.L. & Brand, M.D. (1990). Control of respiration and oxidative phosphorylation in isolated rat liver cells. *European Journal of Biochemistry*, *192*, 355–362.

Calik, P. & Ozdamar, T. H. (2002). Metabolic flux analysis for human therapeutic protein productions and hypothesis for new therapeutical strategies in medicine. *Biotechnol. Eng. J.*, *11*, 49-68.

Camacho, D., de la Fuente, A. & Mendes, P. (2005). The origin of correlations in metabolomics data. *Metabolomics, 1*, 53-63.

Campbell, D.B. (1990). The use of kinetic-dynamic interactions in the evaluation of drugs. *Psychopharmacology*, *100*, 433-450.

Castrillo, J.I., Zeef, L.A., Hoyle, D.C., Zhang, N., Hayes, A., Gardner, D.CJ., Cornell, M.J., Petty, J., Hakes, L., Wardleworth, L., Rash, B., Brown, M., Dunn, W.B., Broadhurst, D., O'Donoghue, K., Hester, S.S., Dunkley, T.PJ., Hart, S.R., Swainston, N., Li, P., Gaskell, S.J., Paton, N.W., Lilley,

K.S., Kell D.B., & Oliver, S.G. (2007). Growth control of the eukaryote cell: a systems biology study in yeast. *Journal of Biology*, *6(4)*, 1-25.

Cerioli, A. & Riani, M. (1999). The ordering of spatial data and the detection of multiple outliers. *J Comput Graph Stat*, *8*, 239-258.

Chappell, M. (1999). Structural identifiability and indistinguishability of certain two-compartment models incorporating nonlinear efflux from the peripheral compartment. *Am. J. Physiol.*, *277*, E481-488.

Chiang, C.L. (1980). An introduction to stochastic processes and their applications; Krieger, Huntington: New York.

Chou, I.C. & Voit, E.O. (2009). Recent developments in parameter estimation and structure identification of biochemical and genomic systems. *Mathematical Biosciences*, *219*, 57-83.

Covertn M.W., Schilling, C.H. & Palsson, B. (2001). Regulation of gene expression in flux balance models of metabolism. *J. Theor. Biol.*, *213*, 73-88.

Crampin, E. J., Schnell, S. & McSharry, P. E. (2004). Mathematical and computational techniques to deduce complex biochemical reaction mechanisms. *Progress in Biophysics & Molecular Biology*, *86*, 77-112.

Cruz-Monteagudo, M., Munteanu, C. R., Borges, F., Cordeiro, M. N., Uriarte, E., Gonzalez-Diaz, H. (2008b). Quantitative Proteome-Property Relationships (QPPRs). Part 1: finding biomarkers of organic drugs with mean Markov connectivity indices of spiral networks of blood mass spectra. *Bioorg Med Chem.*, *16*, 9684-9693.

Cruz-Monteagudo, M., Munteanu, C. R., Borges, F., Cordeiro, M. N. D. S., Uriarte, E., Chou, K. C. & González-Díaz, H., (2008a). Stochastic molecular descriptors for polymers. 4. Study of complex mixtures with topological indices of mass spectra spiral and star networks: The blood proteome case. *Polymer*, *49*, 5575-5587.

Daniel, W. W. (1978). *Applied Nonparametric Statistics*. Houghton Mifflin Co. Boston, Massachussetts, *510*.

Denkert, C., Budczies, J., Weichert, W., Wohlgemuth, G., Scholz, M., Kind, T., Niesporek, S., Noske, A., Buckendahl, A., Dietel, M. & Fiehn, O. (2008). Metabolite profiling of human colon carcinoma – deregulation of TCA cycle and amino acid turnover. *Molecular Cancer*, *7(72)*, 1-15.

Derendorf, H. & Meibohm, B. (1999). Modeling of pharmacokineitc/ pharmacodynamic (PK/PD) relationships: concepts and perspectives. *Pharm. Res.*, *13*, 176-185.

Diaz-Sierra, R., Lozano, J.B. & Fairen, V. (1999). Deduction of chemical mechanisms from the linear response around steady-state. *J. Phys. Chem. A, 103*, 337-343.

Dimitriadou, E., Barth, M., Windischberger, C., Hornik, K. & Moser, E. (2004). A quantitative comparison of functional MRI cluster analysis. *Artif. Intell. Med., 31*, 57-71.

Droesbeke, J. J., Fine, J. & Saporta, G. (1997). *Plans d'expériences: applications à l'entreprise.* Technip: Paris.

Duatre, J. M., Santos, J. B. & Melo, L. C. (1999). Comparison of similarity coefficient based on RAPD markers in the common bean. *Genet. Mol. Biol., 22*, 427-432.

Duineveld, C.A.A.; Smilde, A.K.; Doorhbos, D.A. (1993a). Comparison of experimental designs combining process and mixture variables. Part I. Design construction and theoretical evaluation. *Chemom. Intell. Lab. Syst., 19*, 295-308.

Duineveld, C.A.A.; Smilde, A.K.; Doorhbos, D.A. (1993b). Comparison of experimental designs combining process and mixture variables. Part II. Design evaluation on measured data. *Chemom. Intell. Lab. Syst., 19*, 309-318.

Durot, M., Bourguignon, P.Y. & Schachter, V. (2009). Genome-scalemodels of bacterial metabolism: reconstruction and applications. *FEMS Microbiol. Rev., 33*, 164-190.

Edwards, J.S., Covert, M. & Palsson, B. (2002). Metabolic modelling of microbes: the flux-bala,ce approach. *Environ. Microbiol., 4*, 133-140.

Eide I. (1996). Strategies for Toxicological Evaluation of Mixtures. *Food Chem. Toxicol., 34*, 1147-1149.

Erecinska, M. & Dagani, F. (1990). Relationships between the neuronal sodium/potassium pump and energy metabolism. Effects of K+, Na+, and adenosine triphosphate in isolated brain synaptosomes. *Journal of General Physiology, 95*, 591-616.

Escofier B. & Pagès, J. (1991). Presentation of correspondence analysis and multiple correspondence analysis with the help of examples. *In*: J. Devillers, & W. Karcher (Eds.), *Applied multivariate analysis in SAR and environmental studies.* Kluwer Academic Publishers, Dordrecht, 1-32.

Estrada E. & Bodin, O. (2008). Using network centrality measures to manage landscape connectivity. *Ecol Appl., 18*, 1810-1825.

Estrada, E. (2006). Protein bipartivity and essentiality in the yeast protein-protein interaction network. *Journal of proteome research, 5*, 2177-2184.

Estrada, E. (2007). Point scattering: a new geometric invariant with applications from (nano)clusters to biomolecules. *J Comput Chem., 28,* 767-777.

Ettenhuber, C., Radykewicz, T., Kofer, W., Koop, H. U., Bacher, A. & Eisenreich, W. (2005). Metabolic flux analysis in complex isotopolog space. Recycling of glucose in tobacco plants. *Phytochemistry, 66,* 323-335.

Everitt, B. S. & Dunn, G. (1992). *Applied multivariate data analysis.* Wiley, New York

Everitt, B. S., Landau, S. & Leese, M. (2001). *Cluster Analysis.* Arnold Publishers, London.

Fall, C. P., Marland, E. S., Wagner, J. M. & Tyson, J. J. (2005). *Computation Cell Biology.* Springer-Verlag, NY, *488.*

Fell, D. A. (1996). *Understanding the Control of Metabolism.* Portland Press, London.

Fendt, S.M., Buescher, J.M., Rudroff, F., Picotti, P., Zamboni, N. & Sauer, U. (2010). Tradeoff between enzyme and metabolite efficiency maintains metabolic homeostasis upon perturbations in enzyme capacity. *Molecular Systems Biology, 6:356,* 1-11.

Fernie, A. R., Trethewey, R. N., Krotzky, A. & Willmitzer, L. (2004). Metabolite profiling: from diagnostics to systems biology. *Nat. Rev. Mol. Cell Biol., 5,* 763-769.

Fischer, E., Zamboni, N. & Sauer, U. (2004). High-throughput metabolic flux analysis based on gas chromatography-mass spectrometry derived 13C constraints. *Anal. Biochem., 325,* 308-316.

Filzmoser, P., Garrett, R. G. & Reimann, C. (2005). Multivariate outlier detection in exploration geochemistry. *Comput Geosci, 31,* 579-587.

Follstad, B.D., Balcarcel, R.R., Stephanopoulos, G. & Wang, D.I. (1999). Metabolic flux analysis of hybridoma continuous culture staeady state multiplicity. *Biotechnol. Bioeng., 63,* 675-683.

Förster, J., Gombert, A.K. & Nielsen, J. (2002). A functional genomics approach using metabolomics and in silico pathway analysis. *Biotechnol. Bioeng., 79,* 703-712.

Gambhir, A., Korke, R., Lee, J., Fu, P.C., Europa, A. & Hu, W.S. (2003). Analysis of cellular metabolismof hybridoma cell at distinct physiological states. *J. Biosc. Bioeng., 95,* 317-327.

Gibbons, F. D. & Roth, P. (2002). Judging the quality of gene expression-based clustering methods using gene annotation. *Genome Res., 12,* 1574-1581.

Gillespie, W.R. (1993). Generalized pharmacokinetic modelling for drug with non-linear binding: I. Theoretical framework. *J. Pharmacokinet. Biopharm., 21*, 99-124.

Glajch, J. L., Kirkland, J. J. & Snyder, L. R. (1982). Practical optimisation of solvent selectivity in liquid-solid chromatography using a mixture-design statistical technique. *J. Chromatogr., 238*, 269-280.

Gnanadesikan, R. & Kettenring, J. R. (1972). Robust estimates, residuals, and outlier detection with multiresponse data. *Biometrics, 28*, 81-124.

Gonzalez-Diaz, H. (2008). Quantitative Proteome-Property Relationships (QPPRs). Part 1: finding biomarkers of organic drugs with mean Markov connectivity indices of spiral networks of blood mass spectra. *Bioorg Med Chem., 16*, 9684-9693.

González-Díaz, H., González-Díaz, Y., Santana, L., Ubeira, F. M. & Uriarte, E. (2008). Proteomics, networks and connectivity indices. *Proteomics, 8*, 750-778.

González-Díaz, H., Tenoriob, E., Castañedob, N., Santanaa, L. & Uriarte, E. (2005). 3D QSAR Markov model for drug-induced eosinophilia— theoretical prediction and preliminary experimental assay of the antimicrobial drug G1. *Bioorganic & Medicinal Chemistry, 13*, 1523-1530.

González-Díaz, H., Vilar, S., Santana, L. & Uriarte, E. (2007). Medicinal Chemistry and Bioinformatics – Current Trends in Drugs Discovery with Networks Topological Indices. *Curr Top Med Chem., 7*, 1025-1039.

Gonzalez-Diaz, H., Prado-Prado, F. & Ubeira, F. M. (2008). Predicting antimicrobial drugs and targets with the MARCH-INSIDE approach. *Curr Top Med Chem., 8*, 1676-1690.

Goodacre, R., Vaidynathan, S., Dunn, W. B., et al. (2004). Metabolomics by numbers: acquiring and understanding global metabolite data. *Trends Biotechnol., 22*, 245-252.

Gordon, A. D. (1999). *Classification.* CRC Pr I Llc, Boca Raton.

Greenacre, M. J. (1984). *Theory and applications of correspondence analysis.* Academic Press, London

Greenacre, M. J. (1993). *Correspondence analysis in practice.* Academic Press, London.

Groen, A.K., van Roermund, C.W.T., Vervoorn, R.C., & Tager, J.M. (1986). Control of gluconeogenesis in rat liver cells. Flux control coefficients of the enzymes in the gluconeogenic pathway in the absence and presence of glucagons. *Biochemical Journal, 237*, part 2, 379–389.

Guebel, D.V., Cánovas, M., Torres, N.V. (2009). Model Identification in Presence of Incomplete Information by Generalized Principal Component Analysis: Application to the Common and Differential Responses of *Escherichia coli* to Multiple Pulse Perturbations in Continuous, High-Biomass Density Culture. *Biotechnol. Bioeng.*

Guttorp, P. (1995). *Stochastic Modeling of Scientific Data*, Chapman and Hall, London, Great Britain.

Hafner, R.P., Brown, G.C. & Brand, M.D. (1990). Analysis of the control of respiration rate, phosphorylation rate, proton leak rate and protonmotive force in isolated mitochondria using the 'top-down' approach of metabolic control theory. *European Journal of Biochemistry*, *188*, 313–319.

Hampel, F. R., Ronchetti, E. M., Rousseeuw, P. J. & Stahel, W. (1986). *Robust statistics. The approach based on influence functions*. Wiley, New York.

Hawkins, D. M. (1980). Identification of outliers. Chapman and Hall, London.

Hayashi, K. & Sakamoto, N. (1986). *Dynamic Analysis of Enzyme Systems. An Introduction*. Springer-Verlag, Berlin.

Heikkilä, H.J. (1999). New models for pharmacokinetic data based on generalized Weibull distribution. *Journal of Biopharmaceutical Statistics*, *9*, 89-107.

Heinrich, R. & Schuster, S. (1996). *The Regulation of Cellular Systems*. Chapman & Hall, New York.

Herwig, C. & von Stockar, U. (2002). A small metabolic flux model to identify transient metabolic regulations in Saccharomyces cerevisiae. *Bioprocess Biosyst. Eng.*, *24*, 395-403.

Hill, A.V. (1910). *J. Physiol.*, 40, iv-vvi.

Hofmeyr, J.H.S., Cornish-Bowden, A., Rohwer, J.M. (1993). Taking enzyme kinetics out of control – putting control into regulation. *Eur. J. Biochem.* *212*, 833-837.

Hollman, P.C.H., Gaag, M.V.D., Mengelers, M.J.B., van Trijp, J.M.P., de Vries, J.H.M. & Katan, M.B. (1996). Absorption and disposition kinetics of the dietary antioxidant quercetin in man. *Free Radical Biology & Medicine*, *21*, 703-707.

Holz, M. & Fahr, A. (2001). Compartment Modeling. *Advanced Drug Delivery Reviews*, *48*, 249-264.

Hotelling, H. & Pabst, M. R. (1936). Rank correlation and tests of significance involving no assumption of normality. *Ann. Math. Statist.*, *7*, 29-43.

Hoyland, A. & Rausand, M. (1994). System Reliability Theory. Models and Statistical Methods. Wiley & Sons, New York, 518p.

Hu, C., Lovejoy, W.S. & Shafer, S.L. (1995). Comparison of some control strategies for three-compartment PK/PD models. *J. Anim. Sci.*, *73*, 177-190.

Ishii, N., Robert, M., Nakayama, Y., Kanai, A. & Tomita, M. (2004). Toward large-scale modeling of the microbial cell for computer simulation. *Journal of Biotechnology*, *113*, 281–294.

Ivanciuc, O., Balaban, T. S. & Balaban, A. T. (1993). Chemical graphs with degenerate topological indices based on information on distances. *Journal of Mathematical Chemistry*, *14*, 21-33.

Jaccard, P. (1912). The distribution of the flora in the alpine zone. *New Phytol.*, *11*, 37-50.

Jacobs, J.R. & Williams, E.A. (1993). Algorithm to control "effect compartment" drug concentrations in pharmacokinetic model-driven drug delivery. *J. Pharmacokinet. Biopharm.*, *21*, 689-734.

Jain, A. K., Murty, M. N. & Flynn, P. J. (1999). Data clustering: a review. *ACM Comput.*

Jamshidi, N. & Palsson, B.O. (2008). Top-down analysis of temporal hierarchy in biochemical reaction networks. *PLOS Computational Biology*, *4*, 1-10.

Janga, S. C. & Babu, M. M. (2008). Network-based approaches for linking metabolism with environment. *Genome Biology*, *9*, 239.1-239.5.

Kacser, H. & Burns, J. A. (1973). The control of flux. Symp. *Soc. Exp. Biol.*, *27*, 65-104.

Kell, D. B. (2004). Metabolomics and systems biology: making sense of the soup. *Curr. Opin. Microbiol.*, *7*, 1-12.

Kell, D. B. (2002). Metabolomics and machine learning: explanatory analysis of complex metabolome data using genetic programming to produce simple, robust rules. *Mol. Biol. Rep.*, *29*, 237-241.

Klamt, S., Stelling, J. (2003). Two approaches for metabolic pathway analysis. *Trends Biotechnol.*, 21, 64-69.

Kose, F., Weckwerth, W., Linke, T. & Fiehn, O. (2001). Visualizing plant metabolomic correlation networks using clique-metabolite matrices. *Bioinformatics*, *17*, 1198-1208.

Kotte, O., Zaugg, J.B. & Heinemann, M. (2010). Bacterial adaptation through distributed sensing of metabolic fluxes. *Molecular System Biology*, *6*: 355, 1-9.

Kruckeberg, A.L., Neuhaus, H.E., Feil, R., Gottlieb, L.D. & Stitt, M. (1989). Decreased-activitymutants of phosphoglucose isomerase in the cytosol and chloroplast of Clarkia xantiana. Impact on mass-action ratios and fluxes to sucrose and starch, and estimation of flux control coefficients and elasticity coefficients. *Biochemical Journal, 261*, part 2, 457–467.

Kruger, N. J., Ratcliffe, R. G. & Roscher, A. (2003). Quantitative approaches for analysing fluxes through plant metabolic networks using NMR and stable isotope labelling. *Phytochemistry Reviews, 2*, 17-30.

Lance, G. N. & Williams, W. T. (1967). A general theory of classificatory sorting strategies 1. Hierarchical systems. *Comput. J., 9*, 373-380.

Lange, B.M. (2006). Integrative analysis of metabolic networks: from peaks to flux models? *Curr. Opin. Plant Biol., 9*, 220-226.

Lansky, P. (1996). A stochastic model for circulatory transport in pharmacokinetics. *Math. Biosc., 132*, 141-167.

Lee, J.M, Gianchandani, E.P. & Papin, J. (2006). Flux balance analaysis in the era of metabolomics, *Briefing in Bioinformatics, 7*, 140-150.

Legendre, P. & Legendre, L. (2000). *Numerical Ecology.* Elsevier, Amsterdam, *853*.

Levine, E. & Hwa, T., (2007). Stochastic fluctuations in metabolic pathways. *PNAS, 104*, 9224-9229.

Lewis, G.D., Asnani, A. & Gerszten, R.E. (2008). Application of Metabolomics to Cardiovascular Biomarker and Pathway Discovery. *J. Am. Coll. Cardiol., 52*, 117-123.

Lindon, J. C., Nicholson, J. K. & Holmes, E. (Eds), (2007). *The Handbook of Metabonomics and Metabolomics.* Elsevier, Amsterdam, *561*.

Llaneras, F. & Picó, J. (2007). An interval approach for dealing with flux distributions and elementary modes activity patterns. *J. Theor. Biol., 246*, 290-308.

Llaneras, F. & Picó, J. (2008). Stoichiometric Modelling of Cell Metabolism. *Journal of Bioscience and Bioengineering, 105*, 1-11.

Macheras, P. & Iliadis, A. (2006). Modeling in Biopharmaceutics, Pharmacokinetics and Pharmacodynamics. Homogeneous and Heterogeneous Approaches. Springer, New Cork, 442.

Maharjan, R. P. & Ferenci, T. (2005). Metabolomic diversity in the species *Escherichia coli* and its relationship to genetic population structure. *Metabolomics, 3*, 235-242.

Malarz, K. & Kułakowski, K. (2005). Matrix representation of evolving networks. *Acta Physica Polonica B, 36*, 2523-2536.

Marín-Hernández, A., Rodríguez-Enríquez, S., Vital- González, P.A. et al. (2006). Determining and understanding the control of glycolysis in fast-growth tumor cells: flux control by an over-expressed but strongly product-inhibited hexokinase. *FEBS Journal, 273*, 1975–1988.

Matis, J.H., Wehrly, T.E. & Metzler, M. (1983). On some stochastic formulations and related statistical moments of pharmacokinetics models. *J. Pharmacokinet. Biopharm.*, 11, 77-91.

Matis, J.H. (1988). An introduction to stochastic compartment models in pharmacokinetics. *In*: Pecile, A. & Rescigno, A. (Eds.), *Pharmacokinetics: Mathematical and Statistical Approaches to Metabolism and Distribution of Chemicals and Drugs*, Plennum Press: New York, 1988.

Matis, J.H. & Wehrly, T.E. (1985). On the use of residence time moments in the statistical analysis of age-dependent stochastic compartment systems. *In*: Capasso, V., Grosso, E. & Paveri-Fontana, S.L. (Eds), *Mathematics in Biology and Medicine*, Springer-Verlag, New York, pp. 386-398.

Matis, J.H. & Wehrly, T.E. (1990). Generalized stochastic compartment models with Erlang transit times. *J. Pharmacokinet. Biopharm.*, 18, 589-607.

Matis, J.H. & Kiffe, T.R. (2000). Stochastic Population Models, Springer-Verlag, New York.

Milligan, G. W. (1980). An examination of the effect of six types of error perturbation on

Milligan, W. G. & Cooper, M. C. (1987). Methodology review: clustering methods. *Appl.*

Moreno-Sánchez, R., Saavedra, E., Rodríguez-Enríquez, S. & Olín-Sandoval V. (2008). Metabolic Control Analysis: A Tool for Designing Strategies to ManipulateMetabolic Pathways. *Journal of Biomedicine and Biotechnology*, 2008, 1-30.

Morgan, J. A. & Rhodes, D. (2002). Mathematical Modeling of Plant Metabolic Pathways. *Metabolic Engineering, 4*, 80-89.

Morgenthal, K. Weckwerth, W. & Steuer, R. (2006). Metabolomic networks in plants: transitions from pattern recognition to biological interpretation. *Biosystems, 83*, 108-117.

Morgenthal, K.,Wienkoop, S., Scholz, M., Selbig, J. & Weckwerth, W. (2005). Correlative GC–TOF–MS based metabolite profiling and LC–MS based protein profiling reveal time-related systemic regulation of metabolite–protein networks and improve pattern recognition for multiple biomarker selection. *Metabolomics, 1*, 109-121.

Mortier, F. & Bar-Hen, A. (2004). Influence and sensitivity measures in correspondence analysis. *Statistics, 38*, 207-215.

Motter, A.E., Gulbahce, N., Almaas, E. & Barabási, A.L. (2008). Predicting synthetic rescues in metabolic networks. *Molecular System Biology*, *4*: *168*, 1-10.

McQuen, J. (1967). Some methods for classification and analysis of multivariate observations. *5th Berkeley Symp. on Math. Statistics and Probability*, 281-298.

Mrabet, Y. & Semmar, N. (2010). Mathematical methods to analysis of topology, functional variability and evolution of metabolic systems based on different decomposition concepts. *Current Drug Metabolism*, *11*, 315-341.

Nicholson, J. K., Lindon, J. C. & Holmes, E. (1999). 'Metabonomics': understanding the metabolic responses of living systems to pathophysiological stimuli via multivariate statistical analysis of biological NMR spectroscopic data. *Xenobiotica*, *29*, 1181-1189.

Nolan, R.P., Fenley, A.P. & Lee, K. (2006). Identifiction of distributed metabolic objectives in the hypermetabolic liver by flux and energy balance analysis. *Metab. Eng.*, *8*, 30-45.

Nyberg, G.B., Balcarcel, R.R., Follstad, B.D., Stephanopoulos, G. & Wang, D.I. (1999). Metabolism of peptideamino acids by Chinese hamster ovary cells grown in a complex medium. *Biotechnol. Bioeng.*, *62*, 324-335.

Nyieredy, S. z., Meier, B., Erdelmeier, C. A. J. & Sticher, O. (1985). "PRISMA": A geometrical design for solvent optimization in HPLC. *J. High Resolut. Chromatogr., Chromatogr. Communi.*, *8*, 186-188.

Oliver, S. G., Winson, M. K., Kell, D. B. & Baganz, F. (1998). Systematic functional analysis of the yeast genome. *Trends Biotechnol.*, *16*, 373-378.

Ott, K. H., Aranibar, N., Singh, B. & Stockton, G. W. (2003). Metabonomics classifies pathways affected by bioactive compounds. Artificial neural network classification of NMR spectra of plant extracts. *Phytochemistry*, *62*, 971-985.

Palsson, B. (2000). The challenge of in silico biology. *Nat. Biotechnol.*, *18*, 1147-1150.

Palsson, B.O. (2006). *System biology: properties of reconstructed networks*. Cambridge University Press, New York.

Palsson, B.O., Price, N.D. & Papin, J.A. (2003). Development of network-based pathway definitions: the need to analyze real metabolic networks. *Trends in Biotechnology*, *21*, 195-198.

Papin, J.A., Price, N.D., Edwards, J.S. & Palsson, B.O. (2002). The genome-scale metabolic extreme pathway structure in *Haemophilius influenzae* shows significant network redundancy. *J. Theor. Biol.*, *215*, 67-82.

Papin, J. A., Stelling, J., Price, N. D., Klamt, S., Schuster, S. & Palson, B. O. (2004). Comparison of network-based pathway analysis methods. *Trends Biotechnol., 22*, 400-405.

Papin, J. A., Price, N. D., Wiback, S. J, Fell, D. A. & Palsson, B. O. (2003). Metabolic pathways in the post-genome era. *Trends Biochem. Sci., 28*, 250-258.

Papin, J.A., Price, N.D. & Palsson, B.Ø. (2002). Extreme pathway lengths and reaction participation genome-scale metabolic networks. *Genome Res., 12*, 1889-1900.

Pattarino, F., Marengo, E., Gasco, M. R. & Carpignano, R. (1993). Experimental design and partial least squares in the study of complex mixtures: microemulsions as drug carriers. *Int. J. Pharm., 91*, 157-165.

Pfeiffer T, Sanchez-Valdenebro I, Nuno J, Montero F, Schuster S (1999). METATOOL: for studying metabolic networks. *Bioinformatics, 15*, 251-257.

Piazza, M., Feng, X.J., Rabinowitz, J.D., Rabitz, H. (2008). Diverse metabolic model parameters generate similar methionine cycle dynamics. *Journal of Theoretical Biology, 251*, 628-639.

Pierens, G.K., Palframan, M.E., Tranter, C.J., Carroll, A.R. & Quinn, R.J. (2005). A robust clustering approach for NMR spectra of natural product extacts. *Magn. Reson. Chem., 43*, 359-365.

Piotrovskii, V.K. (1987). Pharmacokinetic stochastic model with Weibull-distributed residence times of drug molecules in the body. *Eur. J. Clin. Pharmacol., 32*, 515-523.

Piotrovskij, V & Van Peer, A. (1998). A model with separate hepatoportal compartment ('first-pass' model): fitting to plasma concentration-time profiles in humans. *J. Pharm. Sci., 87*, 470-481.

Ponce, Y. M. (2004). Total and local (atom and atom type) molecular quadratic indices: significance interpretation, comparison to other molecular descriptors, and QSPR/QSAR applications. *Bioorganic & Medicinal Chemistry, 12*, 6351-6369. *Psych Meas., 11*, 329-354.

Poolman, M.G., Fell, D.A. & Raines, C.A. (2003). Elementary modes analysis of photosynthate metabolism in the chloroplast stroma. *FEBS J., 270*, 430-439.

Poolman, M.G., Assmus, H.E. & Fell, D.A. (2004). Applications of metabolic modelling to plant metabolism. *Journal of Experimental Botany, 55*, 1177-1186.

Price, N.D., Papin, J.A. & Palsson, B.O. (2002). Determination of redundancy and systems properties of the metabolic network of Heliobacter pylori using genome-scale extreme pathway analysis. *Genome Res., 12*, 760-769.

Price, N.D., Papin, J.A., Schilling, C.H. & Palsson, B.O. (2003). Genome-scale microbial in silico models: the constraints-based approach. *Trends Biotechnol., 21*, 162-169.

Price, N.D., Reed, J.L. & Palsson, B.O. (2004). Genome-scale models of microbial cells: evaluating the consequences of constraints. *Nature Reviews. Microbiology, 2*, 886-897.

Provost, A. & Bastin, G. (2004). Dynamic metabolic modelling under the balanced growth condition. *Journal of Process Control, 14*, 717-728.

Purdue, P. (1979). *In*: Matis, J.H., Patten, B.C. & White, G.C. (Eds.). *Compartmental Analysis of Ecosystem Models.*, Int. Coop Publ. House, Fairland, MD.

Purdue, P. (1974). Stochastic theory of compartments: One and two compartment systems. *Bull. Math. Biol., 36*, 577-587.

Ralser, M., Wamelink, M.M., Kowald, A., Gerisch, B., Heeren, G., Struys, E.A., Klipp, E., Jakobs, C., Breitenbach, M., Lehrach, H. & Krobitsch, S. (2007). Dynamic rerouting of the carbohydrate flux is key to counteracting oxidative stress. *Journal of Biology, 6* (10), 1-18.

Ratcliffe, R.G. & Shachar-Hill, Y. (2006). Measuring multiple fluxes through plant metabolic networks. *Plant J., 45*, 490-511.

Resendis-Antonio, O., Reed, J.L, Encarnación, S., Collado-Vides, J. & Palsson, B. Ø. (2007). Metabolic Reconstruction and Modeling of Nitrogen Fixation in *Rhizobium etli. PLoS Comput. Biol.*, 3(10), 1887-1895.

Ritschel, W.A., Kearn, G.L (1999). Handbook of Basic Pharmacokinetics, 5th ed.; *American Pharmaceutical Association*, Washington, D.C.

Robinson, R. B. (2005). Identifying outliers in correlated water quality data. *J Environ Eng, 134*, 651-657.

Rockafellar, R.T. (1970). *Convex analysis*. Princeton University Press, Princeton.

Rodríguez-Enríquez, S., Torres-Márquez, M.E. & Moreno-Sánchez, R. (2000). "Substrate oxidation and ATP sypply in AS-30D hepatoma cells," *Archives of Biochemistry and Biophysics, 375*, 21–30.

Rodriguez, A. & Infante, S. (2009). Network models in the study of metabolism. *Electronic Journal of Biotechnology, 12*(3), 1-19.

Roessner, U., Luedemann, A., Brust, D., et al., (2001). Metabolic profiling allows comprehensive phenotyping of genetically or environmentally modified plant systems. *Plant Cell, 13*, 11-29.

Rousseeuw, P. J. & Leroy, A. M. (1987). Robust regression and outlier detection. Wiley, New York.

Rousseeuw, P. J. & Van Zomeren, B. C. (1990). Unmasking multivariate outliers and leverage points. *J Am Stat Assoc, 85*, 633-651.

Rouvray, D. H. (1992). The definition and role of similarity concepts in the chemical and physical sciences. *J. Chem. Inf. Comput. Sci., 32*, 580-586.

Roux, M. (1991a). Basic Procedures in hierarchical cluster analysis. In: *Applied Multivariate Analysis in SAR and Environmental Studies*, Devillers, J. and Karcher, W. Eds. Kluwer Academic Publishers, Dordrecht, 115-136.

Roux, M. (1991b). Interpretation of hierarchical clustering. In: *Applied Multivariate Analysis in SAR and Environmental Studies*, Devillers, J. and Karcher, W. Eds. Kluwer Academic Publishers, Dordrecht, 137-152.

Sado, G. & Sado, M. Chr. (1991). *Les plans d'expériences, de l'expérimentation à l'assurance qualité* ; Afnor technique, Paris.

Savageau, M. A. (1976). *Biochemical Systems Analysis*. Addison-Wesley, Reading, MA.

Scheffe, H. (1958). *J. R. Stat. Soc.* B, *20*, 344.

Scheffe, H. (1963). *J. R. Stat. Soc.* B, *25*, 235.

Schilling, C.H., Palsson, B.O. (2000). Assessment of the metabolic capabilities of *Haemophilius influenzae* Rd through a genome-scale pathway analysis. *J. Theor. Biol., 203*, 249-283.

Schilling, C.H., Schuster, S., Palsson, B.O. & Heinrich, R. (1999) Metabolic pathway analysis: basic concepts and scientific applications in the post-genomic era. *Biotechnol. Prog., 15*, 296–303.

Schilling C.H., Letscher D, Palsson B.O. (2000). Theory for the systemic definition of metabolic pathways and their use in interpreting metabolic function from a pathway-oriented perspective. *J Theor Biol 203*,229–248.

Schilling, C.H., Covert, M.W., Famili, I., Church, G.M., Edwards, J.S. & Palsson, B.O. (2002). Genome-scale metabolic model of Heliobacter pylori 26695. *J. Bacteriol., 184,* 4582-4593.

Schilling, C. H., Edwards, J. S., Letscher, D. & Palsson, B. (2001). Combining pathway analysis with flux balance analysis for the comprehensive study of metabolic systems. *Biotechnol Bioeng, 71*, 286-306.

Schimizu, H. (2002). Metabolic engineering– integrating methodologies of molecular breeding and bioprocess systems engineering. *J. Biosc. Bioeng.*, *94*, 563-573.

Schmidt, K., Nielsen, J. & Villadsen, J. (1999). Quantitative analysis of metabolic fluxes in Escherichia coli, using two-dimensional NMR spectroscopy and complete isotopomer models. *J. Biotechnol.*, *71*, 175-189.

Schuetz R, Kuepfer L, Sauer U (2007) Systematic evaluation of objective functions for predicting intracellular fluxes in *Escherichia coli*. *Mol. Syst. Biol. 3*,1–15

Schuster, S., Hilgetag, C. (1994). On elementary flux modes in biochemical reaction systems at stedy-state. *J. Biol. Syst.*, *2*, 165-182.

Schuster, S., Dandekar, T., Fell, D.A. (1999). Detection of elementary flux modes in biochemical networks: a promising tool for pathway analysis and metabolic engineering. *Trends Biotechnol.*, *17*, 53-60.

Schuster S, Pfeiffer T, Moldenhauer F, Koch I, Dandekar T (2002a). Exploring the pathway structure of metabolism: decomposition into subnetworks and application to Mycoplasma pneumoniae. *Bioinformatics*, *18*, 351-361

Schuster S, Hilgetag C, Woods JH, Fell DA (2002b) Reaction routes in biochemical reaction systems: algebraic properties, validated calculation procedure and example from nucleotide metabolism. *J Math Biol*, *45*, 153-181

Schwender, J., Ohlrogge, J. & Shachar-Hill, Y. (2004). Understanding flux in plant metabolic networks. *Curr. Opin. Plant Biol.*, *7*, 309-317.

Seber, G. A. F. (1984). Multivariate observations. Wiley, New York.

Seber, G.A.F. & Wild, C.J. (1989). Nonlinear Regression. Wiley, New York.

Semmar, N., Jay, M. & Chemli, R. (2001). Chemical diversification trends in *Astragalus caprinus* (Leguminosae) based on the flavonoid pathway. *Biochemical Systematics and Ecology*, *29,* 727-738.

Semmar, N., Bruguerolle, B., Boullu-Ciocca, S. & Simon, N. (2005b). Cluster analysis: an alternative method for covariate selection in population pharmacokinetic modeling. *Journal of Pharmacokinetics and Pharmacodynamics*, *32, 333-358.*

Semmar, N., Jay, M., Farman, M. & Chemli, R. (2005a). Chemotaxonomic analysis of *Astragalus caprinus* (Fabaceae) based on the flavonic patterns. *Biochemical Systematics and Ecology*, *33*, 187-200.

Semmar, N., Jay, M. & Nouira, S. (2007). A new approach to graphical and numerical analysis of links between plant chemotaxonomy and secondary metabolism from HPLC data smoothed by a simplex mixture design. *Chemoecology*, *17*, 139-156.

Semmar, N. & Simon, N. (2006). Review in pharmacokinetic models on corticosteroids. *Mini Reviews in Medicinal Chemistry*, 6, 109-120.

Semmar, N., Urien, S., Bruguerolle, B. & Simon, N. (2008). Independent-model diagnostics for a priori identification and interpretation of outliers from a full pharmacokinetic database: correspondence analysis, Mahalanobis distance and Andrews curves. *J Pharmacokinet Pharmacodyn, 35*, 159-183.

Semmar, N. (2010). A New Mixture Design-Based Approach to Graphical Screening of Potential Interconnections and Variability Processes in Metabolic Systems. *Chem. Biol & Drug Design* 75, 91-105.

Serge, D., Vitkup, D., Church, G.M. (2002) Analysis of optimality in natural and perturbed metabolic networks. *PNAS*, *99*, 15112–15117.

Shannon, C. E. (1948). A mathematical theory of communication. *Bell System Tech. J., 27*, 379.

Shargel, L. & Yu, A. (1999). *Applied Biopharmaceutics & Pharmacokinetics*. McGraw-Hill, New York., *768*.

Sharma, N.S., Ierapetritou, M.G. & Yarmush, M.L. (2005). Novel quantitative tools for engineering analysis of hepatocyte cultures in bioartificial liver systems. *Biotechnol. Bioeng.*, *92*, 321-335.

Smallbone, K., Simeonidis, E., Broomhead, D.S. & Kell, D.B. (2007). Something from nothing—bridging the gap between constraint-based and kinetic modelling. *FEBS Journal*, *274*, 5576-5585.

Smith, C.E., Lansky, P. & Lung, T.H. (1997). Cycle-time ana residence-time density approximations in a stochastic model for circulatory transport. *Bull.Math.Biol.*, *59*, 1-22.

Sorribas, A., Lozano, J.B. & Fairen, V. (1998). Deriving chemical and biochemical model networks from experimental measurements. *Recent Res. Devel. in Physical Chem.*, *2*, 553-573.

Spearman, C. (1904). The proof and measurement of association between two thing. *Amer. J. Psychol., 15*, 72-101.

Sprott, J.C. (2003). *Chaos and Time-Series Analysis*. Oxford University Press, Oxford.

Sriram, G., Fulton, D.B., Iyer, V.V., Peterson, J.M., Zhou, R., Westgate, M.E., Spalding, M.H. & Shanks, J.V. (2004). Quantification of Compartmented Metabolic Fluxes in Developing Soybean Embryos by Employing Biosynthetically Directed Fractional 13C Labeling, Two-Dimensional

[^{13}C, ^{1}H] Nuclear Magnetic Resonance, and Comprehensive Isotopomer Balancing. *Plant Physiology*, *136*, 3043-3057.

Stelling, J. (2004). Mathematical models in microbial systems biology. *Current Opinion in Microbiology, 7*, 513-518.

Stelling, J., Klamt, S., Bettenbrock, K., Schuster, S. & Gilles, E.D. (2002). Metabolic network structure determines key aspects of functionality and regulation. *Nature*, *420*, 190-193.

Stephanopoulos, G.N., Aristidou, A.A. & Nielsen, J. (1998). *Metabolic engineering: principles and methodologies*. Academic Press, San Diego.

Steuer, R. (2006). On the analysis and interpretation of correlations in metabolomic data. *Briefings in Bioinformatics, 7*, 151-158.

Steuer, R., Gross, T. Selbig, J. & Blasius, B. (2006). Structural kinetic modeling of metabolic networks. *PNAS*, *103*, 11868-11873.

Steuer, R. (2007). Computational approaches to the topology, stability and dynamics of metabolite networks. *Phytochemistry, 68*, 2139-2151.

Steuer, R., Nesi, A.N., Fernie, A.R., Gross, T., Blasius, B. & Selbig, J. (2007). From structure to dynamics of metabolic pathways: application to the plant mitochondrial TCA cycle. *Bioinformatics*, *23*, 1378-1385.

Steuer, R., Kurths, J., Fiehn, O., Weckwerth, W. (2003a). Interpreting correlations in metabolic networks. *Biochem. Soc. Trans., 31(6)*, 1476-1478.

Steuer, R., Kurths, J., Fiehn, O. & Weckwerth, W. (2003b). Observing and interpreting correlations in metabolomic networks. *Bioinformatics, 19(8)*, 1019-1026.

Strang, G. (1986). *Introduction to Applied Mathematics*. Wellesley-Cambridge Press, Wellesley, M.A., 665-672.

Strogatz, S.H. (2000). *Nonlinear Dynamic and Chaos*. Westview Press, Cambridge.

Sumner, L. W., Mendes, P., Dixon, R. A. (2003). Plant metabolomics: large-scale phytochemistry in the functional genomics era. *Phytochemistry, 62*, 817-836.

Swaroop, R. & Winter, W. R. (1971). A statistical technique for computer identification of outliers in multivariate data. *NASA Tech Notes* D-6472.

Sweetlove, L. J. & Fernie, A. R. (2005). Regulation of metabolic networks: understanding metabolic complexity in the systems biology era. *New Phytol., 168*, 9-24.

Takiguchi, N., Shimizu, H. & Shioya, S. (1997). An on-line physiological state recognition system for the lysine fermentation process based on a metabolic reaction model. *Biotechnol. Bioeng., 55*, 170-181.

Tamir, A. (Ed.), 1998. *Applications of Markov Chains in Chemical Engineering*. Elsevier, Amsterdam, *604*.

Tikunov, Y., Lommen, A., Ric de Vos, C.H. , Verhoeven, H.A., Bino, R.J., Hall, R.D. & Bovy, A.G. (2005). A Novel Approach for Nontargeted Data Analysis for Metabolomics. Large-Scale Profiling of Tomato Fruit Volatiles. *Plant Physiology, 139*, 1125-1137.

Tiziani, S., Lodi, A., Khanim, F.L., Viant, M.R., Bunce, C.M., Günther, U.L. (2009). Metabolomic Profiling of Drug Responses in Acute Myeloid Leukaemia Cell Lines. *PLoS ONE, 4*, 1-10.

Todeschini, R. & Consonni, V. (2000). *Handbook of Molecular Descriptors*: Wiley-VCH.

Trinh, C.T., Wlaschin, A., Srienc, F. (2009). Elemenary mode analysis: a useful metabolic pathway analysis tool for characterizing cellular metabolism. *Appl. Microbiol. Biotechnol., 81*, 813-826.

Tuljapurkar, S. & Cawell, H. (1997). *Structured-population models in marine, terrestrial, and freshwater systems*. Chapman & Hall, New York.

Van-Dien, S.J., Iwatani, S., Usuda, Y. & Matsui, K. (2006). Theoretical analysis of amino acid-producing *Escherichia coli* using a stoichiometric model and multivariate linear regression. *J. Biosc. Bioeng., 102*, 34-40.

Van Rossum, J.M., de Bie, J.G.M., van Lingen, G. & Teeuwen W.A. (1989). Pharmacokinetics from a dynamical system point of view. *J. Pharmacokin. Biopharmacol., 17*, 365-397.

Varma A. & Palsson, B.O. (1994). Stoichiometric Flux Balance Models Quantitatively Predict Growth and Metabolic By-Product Secretion in Wild-Type *Escherichia coli* W3110. *Applied and Environmental Microbiology*, 60, 3724-3731.

Veflingstad, S.R., Almeida, J., Voit, E.O. (2004). Priming nonlinear searches for pathway identification. *Theoretical Biology and Medical Modelling, 1(8)*, 1-14.

Veng-Pedersen, P. (2001). Noncompartmentally-based pharmacokinetic modelling. *Advanced Drug Delivery Reviews, 48*, 265-300.

Vilar, S., Estrada, E., Uriarte, E., Santana, L. & Gutierrez, Y. (2005). In silico studies toward the discovery of new anti-HIV nucleoside compounds through the use of TOPS-MODE and 2D/3D connectivity indices. 2. Purine derivatives. *Journal of chemical information and modeling, 45*, 502-514.

Wagner, C. & Urbanczik, R. (2005). The Geometry of the Flux Cone of a Metabolic Network. *Biophysical Journal, 89*, 3837-3845.

Waite, S. (2000). *Statistical Ecology in Practice*. Prentice Hall, Harlow, *414*.

Wanders, R. J., Groen, R. J., van Roermund, R. J. & Tager, J. M. (1984). Factors determining the relative contribution of the adenine-nucleotide translocator and the ADP-regenerating system to the control of oxidative phosphorylation in isolated rat-liver mitochondria. *European Journal of Biochemistry, 142*, 417–424.

Ward, J. H. (1963). Hierarchical grouping to optimize an objective function. *J. Am. Stat. Assoc., 58*, 236-244.

Weckwerth, W. (2003). Metabolomics in Systems Biology. *Annu. Rev. Plant Biol., 54*, 669-689.

Weckwerth, W., Loureiro, M., Wenzel, K., Fiehn, O. (2004a). Differential metabolic networks unravel the effects of silent plant phenotypes. *Proc. Natl. Acad. Sci., U.S.A., 101*, 7809-7814.

Weckwerth, W., Wenzel, K. & Fiehn, O. (2004b). Process for the integrated extraction, identification and quantification of metabolites, proteins and RNA to reveal their co-regulation in biochemical networks. *Proteomics, 4(1)*, 78-83.

Weckwerth, W. & Morgenthal, K. (2005). Metabolomics: from pattern recognition to biological interpretation. *Drug Discovery Today: Targets, 10 (22)*, 1551-1558.

Weiss, M., (1984). A note on the role of generalized inverse Gaussian distribution of circulatory transit times in pharmacokinetics. *J. Math. Biol., 20*, 95-102.

Weiss, M. (1983). Use of Gamma distributed residence times in pharmacokinetics. *Eur. J. Clin. Pharmacol., 25*, 695-702.

Welling, P.G. 1997. *Pharmacokinetics: Processes, Mathematics and Applications*. American Chemical Society, Washington, DC, *393*.

Wiback, S.J. & Palsson, B.O. (2002). Extreme Pathway Analysis of Human Red Blood Cell Metabolism. *Biophysical Journal, 83*, 808-818.

Wienkoop, S., Morgenthal, K., Wolschin, F. & Scholz, M. (2008). Integration of Metabolomic and Proteomic Phenotypes. *Molecular & Cellular Proteomics, 7.9*, 1725-1736.

Wildermuth, M.C. (2000). Metabolic control analysis: biological applications and insights. *Genome Biology, 1(6)*, 1-5.

Williams, T. C. R., Miguet, L., Masakapalli, S. K., Kruger, N. J., Sweetlove, L. J. & Ratcliffe, R. G. (2008). Metabolic Network Fluxes in Heterotrophic Arabidopsis Cells: Stability of the Flux Distribution under Different Oxygenation Conditions. *Plant Physiology, 148*, 704-718.

Wimmer, G., Didík, L., Michal, M., Mudríkova, A. & Ďurišová, M. (1999). Numerical simulation of stochastic circulatory models. *Bull. Math. Biol.*, *61*, 365-377.

Wishart, D.S. (2007). Current progress in computational metabolomics. *Briefings in Bioinformatics, 8*, 279-293.

Wu, L., van Winden, W.A., van Gulik, W.M. & Heijnen, J.J. (2005) Application of metabolome data in functional genomics: A conceptual strategy. *Metabolic Engineering, 7*, 302–310.

Yanai, I., Baugh, L. R., Smith, J. J., Roehrig, C., Shen-Orr, S. S., Claggett, J. M., Hill, A. A., Slonim, D. K. & Hunter, C. P. (2008). Pairing of competitive and topologically distinct regulatory modules enhances patterned gene expression. *Molecular Systems Biology, 4(163)*, 1-12.

Yang, C.R., Shapiro, B.E., Mjolsness, E.D. & Hatfield, G.W. (2005). An enzyme mechanism langage for the mathematical modeling of metabolic pathways. *Bioinformatics, 21*, 774-780.

Yang, T. H., Wittmann, C. & Heinzle, E. (2004). Metabolic network simulation using logical loop algorithm and Jacobian matrix. *Metabolic Engineering, 6*, 256-267.

Yang, Y.T., Bennett, G.N. & San K.Y. (1998). Genetic and metabolic engineering. Electronic Journal of Biotechnology, 1 (3), 134-141.

Yetukuri, L., Katajamaa, M., Medina-Gomez, G., Seppänen-Laakso, T., Vidal-Puig, A. & Matej Orešič (2007). Bioinformatics strategies for lipidomics analysis: characterization of obesity related hepatic steatosis. *BMC System Biology, 1:12*, 1-15.

Yugi, K., Nakayama, Y., Kinoshita, A. & Tomita, M. (2005). Hybrid dynamic/static method for large-scale simulation of metabolism. *Theoretical Biology and Medical Modelling, 2(42)*, 1-11.

Zar, J. H. (1999). *Biostatistical Analysis.* Prentice Hall, New Jersey, *663*.

Zhen, Y., Krausz, K.W., Chen, C., Idle, J.R., & Gonzalez, F.J. (2007). Metabolomic and Genetic Analysis of Biomarkers for Peroxisome Proliferator-Activated Receptor α Expression and Activation. *Molecular Endocrinology, 21*, 2136-2151.

Zhong, J.J. (2002). Plant cell culture for production of paclitaxel and other taxanes. *J. Biosc. Bioeng., 94*, 591-599.

Zu, X. L. & Guppy, M. (2004). Cancer metabolism: facts, fantasy, and fiction". *Biochemical and Biophysical Research Communications, 313*, 459–465.

Index

C

D

E

N

O

S